Neuroscience Research Progress

nova
Medicine & Health
New York

Neuroscience Research Progress

New Perspectives in Neuroscience
Prachi Srivastava, PhD (Editor)
Neha Srivastava, PhD (Editor)
Prekshi Garg (Editor)
2022. ISBN: 978-1-68507-754-9 (Softcover)
2022. ISBN: 978-1-68507-847-8 (eBook)

Psychobiological Principles of the Memory Process
Ignacio González-Burgos, PhD
2022. ISBN: 978-1-68507-661-0 (Hardcover)
2022. ISBN: 978-1-68507-769-3 (Softcover)

The Dentate Gyrus: Structure, Functions and Health Implications
Feng-Ru Tang, PhD, MD (Editor)
2021. ISBN: 978-1-68507-212-4 (Hardcover)
2021. ISBN: 978-1-68507-240-7 (eBook)

Systemic, Cellular and Molecular Mechanisms of Physiological Functions and Their Disorders (Proceedings of I. Beritashvili Center for Experimental Biomedicine – 2021)
Nargiz Nachkebia, PhD (Editor)
Nodar P. Mitagvaria, PhD, Dr. of Sci. (Editor)
2021. ISBN: 978-1-68507-113-4 (Hardcover)
2021. ISBN: 978-1-68507-135-6 (eBook)

Neuromanagement: Neuroscience for Organizations
Michela Balconi (Editor)
2021. ISBN: 978-1-53619-562-0 (Hardcover)
2021. ISBN: 978-1-53619-650-4 (eBook)

More information about this series can be found at
https://novapublishers.com/product-category/series/neuroscience-research-progress/

Franco F. Orsucci and Nicoletta Sala
Editors

Neuroscience and Technology Transform the Educational Ecosystem

nova
Medicine & Health
New York

DOI: https://doi.org/10.52305/NHNG6007

Library of Congress Cataloging-in-Publication Data

ISBN: 979-8-88697-157-6

Published by Nova Science Publishers, Inc. † New York

Contents

Preface

Neuroscience is exciting. Understanding how thoughts work, how connections are made, how the memory works, how we process information, how information is stored - it's all fascinating.

Lisa Randall

Scientists, educationalists and policymakers are increasingly recognizing the relevance of neuroscience to education and its potential impact on pedagogy. Our thoughts, perceptions and actions continuously change the strength of connections between neurons in the brain. These physical connections represent our understanding and knowledge of the world around us, our brain plasticity. Education plays a crucial role in changing brains. Teachers are the professionals changing brain connectivity in young people daily! At the same time, significant neuroscience insights reveal the impact of environmental factors of all human technology interfaces on the brain.

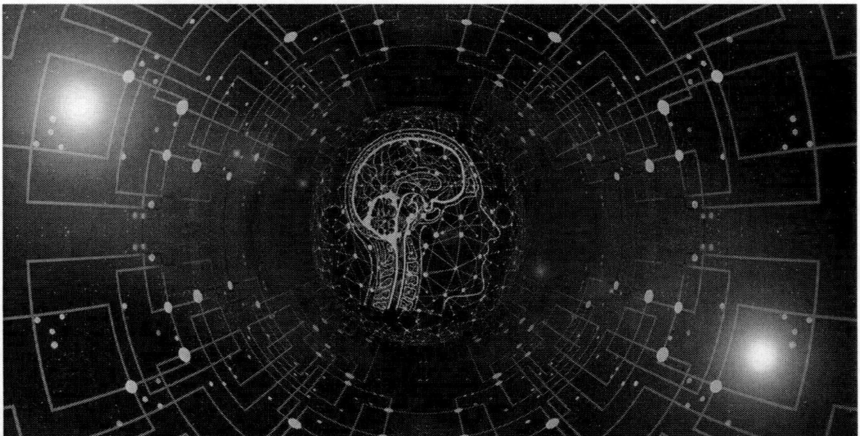

(image free reproduction)

Human interfaces, social media, videogaming and animation play an exponentially growing role in active learning in and out of the classroom. Beyond Froebel and Montessori, kindergarten is potentially now everywhere, for all learning ages. With advances in neuroscience and educational technology, student learning can reach new frontiers. Rather than a default learning model, there is now a fluidity in the way educators of all kinds can deliver content, interact with students, take on feedback, and modify their teaching approach. Students have access to seamless e-learning experiences influenced by psychology and the latest research on how the brain works. Learning has changed remarkably with these advances in and out of the classroom forever. Learning becomes more fun and more social. Games with features like rewards, advice, and feedback increase motivation. If students are motivated, they are likely to stay at a task or practice a skill longer. This kind of immersive learning also feeds into the science of brain plasticity.

By offering broader and more interactive EdTech experiences that stimulate the entire sensory nervous system and allow for many challenges and opportunities to practice, students of any age can build on their neuroplasticity through diverse learned experiences. It is an e-learning revolution! Neuroscience and educational technology have reshaped the way learning is delivered and revolutionized the way we think about education. Learning becomes a highly personalized process building stronger minds, more expansive neural pathways, and individuals with love for lifelong education. Educators can take a dynamic, data-driven approach that challenges students to think critically, solve socially, and diversify how their learning occurs. Students of all ages can transform from passive learners into active engagers who take control of their evolutionary pathways.

Book Organization

This book is divided in three sections.

Section 1. "**Theory**" contains important chapters dedicated to the neuroscience, some of which have already appeared on the International journal *Chaos and Complexity Letters* in the past fifteen years, but their importance suggested to the editors to repropose them in this book.

In the first chapter *"Interdisciplinary knowledge and beyond: algorithms and patterns"* (published on CCL 13 issue 1 pp. 1-13) Franco Orsucci opens this special number exploring in a non-formal way the impact of interdisciplinary knowledge on specialised disciplines. The author considers the epistemological and pedagogical implications.

Walter J. Freeman in "*Indirect Biological Measures of Consciousness from Field Studies of Brains as Dynamical Systems*" (published on CCL 4 issue 3 pp. 33-52) proposes that consciousness can be defined as a field of force that is centered in a brain and that operates through the body simultaneously into all levels of the surround from subatomic to social.

Qinye Tong, Lunping Fang, Hong Zhang, Mingqi Qian, Xu Li and Xiaobeng Han in "*Circle Mapping Applied in Neural Impulse Sequence Analysis—neuron code research*" (CCL 4 issue 2 pp. 205-220) confirm that the neural impulse sequence is neural information coding, answering the following questions: (1) Is the neural impulse sequence space an ordered space? (2) Are there any features of operation or mapping in the neural impulse sequence space?

Evguenia V. Liutikova presents "*Cognitive Axioms as Low-Level Rules of Communicative and Other Practices in Social Dynamical Systems*" (published on CCL 4 issue 1 pp. 57-76) describes research data in basic social cognition forms - attitudes, beliefs, stereotypes, prejudices, social representations - providing for treating these mental foundations of social cognition and behaviour as having a common principal function of cognitive axioms in perceiving, interpreting, and applying information to social practises.

Franco Orsucci in "*Mind Force Theory: hyper-network dynamics in neuroscience*" (published on CCL 4 issue 3 pp. 9-32) presents the importance of the application of hyper-network dynamics in the field of the neuroscience.

Walter J. Freeman "*On the Nature and Neural Mechanisms of Mind Force*" (published on CCL 6 issue 1-2, pp. 7-15) describes the mind that is the structure of the activity of the brain. Mind is then expressed in the intentional behavior that is controlled by the forces exerted by the brain activity on the sensory and motor input/output systems of the brain.

Frederick David Abraham in "*An Inquiry/Review into the Generalized Spectrum of Dimensions, D_q, and its Relevance to Research*" (published CCL vol. 4 issue 2 pp, 193-204) describes the generalized spectrum of dimensions of time series which provides additional measures of a signal that single dimensional measures fail to offer.

Harriet W. Hanlon and John Docker in "*Gender-Specific Strange Attractors Describe Human Brain Development During Childhood, Latency, Adolescence and Young Adulthood*" (published on CCL vol. 4 issue 2 pp. 221-256). The study confirms that brain regions do not develop concurrently and that each sex has different critical periods for assimilating the culture in hunter/gatherer and complex-reasoning networks.

Section 2. is "**Technology**" that collects the works that describe the connection between neuroscience, technology and education.

Nicoletta Sala in "*Extended Reality in Education*" presents a brief overview of the use of extended reality (XR, which comprises virtual reality, augmented reality, and mixed reality) in education.

Raimondo Sgrò *in "Educational Robotic In Learning Path"* describes the importance of the robotics and the games in the leaning path.

Nicoletta Sala in "*Fractal Geometry in Computer Graphics and Virtual Reality*" (paper just published on CCL vol. 3, issue 2, pp. 153 – 168) presents the fractal geometry as a tool to create virtual worlds using techniques of computer graphics.

Section 3. is "**Case Study**" where Laura Cancellara, Nicoletta Sala, Paola Appeddu, Alessandro Lai and Franco Orsucci present an Italian research project in the chapter titled: "*Multidisciplinary Skills in the School of Complexity: Educational Technologies, Human Factor & Non Cognitive Skills*". It involves new technology, non cognitive skills, and new educational approaches in the teaching environment.

London, 10 April 2022

Franco Orsucci and Nicoletta Sala
Book Editors

Section 1. Theory

Chapter 1

Interdisciplinary Knowledge and Beyond: Algorithms and Patterns*

Franco F. Orsucci†
University College London, NCI University London, UK

> We are not students of some subject matter, but students of problems. Problems might cut right across the boundaries of any subject matter or discipline.
>
> Karl Popper

Abstract

Throughout history, scientists and philosophers have defined disciplines in different ways. An influential tradition is taking the view that disciplines are tools for dealing with real world problems and scientists are not students of some subject matter, but students of problems. Some disciplines can be flexible and more adaptable to the nature of problems, as for example mathematics. Aristotle argued that also physics, biology and psychology can be considered as flexible to the nature and properties of their matter. However, the last century has seen an explosion of scientific specialisations, sometimes as micro-tools for local problems, sometimes as micro academic domains for university administration. The last decades have seen interdisciplinary emergence as a counter-force of problem focused collaborations. This process has seen highly dynamical landscapes of interdisciplinary collaborations, with different degrees

---

* This article was originally published in Chaos and Complexity Letters, volume 13 number 1 (2019).

† Corresponding Author's Email: f.orsucci@ucl.ac.uk.

In: Neuroscience and Technology Transform the Educational Ecosystem
Editors: Franco F. Orsucci and Nicoletta Sala
ISBN: 979-8-88697-157-6

from interaction to fusion between disciplines. We explore in a non-formal way the impact of interdisciplinary knowledge on specialised disciplines. We consider the epistemological and pedagogical implications.

1. Throughout history, scientists and philosophers have defined disciplines in different ways. An influential tradition is taking the view that disciplines are tools for dealing with real world problems and scientists are not "students of some subject matter, but students of problems" (Popper, 1968, 1974). Some disciplines can be flexible and more adaptable to the nature of problems, as for example mathematics. Aristotle argued that also physics, biology and psychology can be considered as flexible to the nature and properties of their matter.

However, the last century has seen an explosion of scientific specializations, sometimes as micro-tools for local problems, sometimes as micro academic domains for university administration (Menken & Keestra, 2016).

The last decades have seen interdisciplinarity's emergence as a counterforce of problem focused collaborations. This process has seen highly dynamical landscapes of interdisciplinary collaborations, with different degrees from interaction to fusion between disciplines. A possible definition might be: "[Interdisciplinary studies is] a process of answering a question, solving a problem, or addressing a topic that is too broad or complex to be dealt with adequately by a single discipline or profession . . . and draws on disciplinary perspectives and integrates their insights through construction of a more comprehensive perspective" (Klein & Newell, 1997).

2. A definition of what interdisciplinarity is deals also with defining our epistemology, in science and everyday life. Boundaries between disciplines are changing depending from the tools and focus we use to observe and define reality. Historically, they have changed many times and they will keep changing. The idea of interdisciplinarity is educative for the very reason that it is innately ambiguous and easily adapted to different times and cultures. In the inherently infinite nature of this approach, a new cohesion has begun to emerge. The prospect of a theory of interdisciplinarity has coalesced around the concepts of integration and complexity (Orsucci, 1998, 2002). Each discipline, after a while, exists in virtue of its own technical language, or jargon. The boundary work of interdisciplinarity is directed into the activity of integration, which is negotiated, situational, and contingent. Therefore, it

includes semantic maps and translations between disciplinary jargons. This will imply transcending local ways of thinking but also the risk of misunderstandings, common in every translational procedure.

Interdisciplinarity entails not only the interpenetration of disciplinary boundaries, but also more fundamentally, a meta-cognitive rethinking of the ways in which we structure knowledge itself (Newell, 1998). However, as Klein (1996) suggests, the interdisciplinary approach to epistemology is not reductionist, nor does it seek a grand unification of transdisciplinary truth claims. Rather, interdisciplinarity shifts epistemology "from absolute answers and solutions to tentativeness and reflexivity. In all interdisciplinary activities, time should be devoted to examining the philosophical underpinnings of the challenge they pose to disciplinary approaches. Good interdisciplinary work requires a strong degree of epistemological reflexivity" (p. 214). Mansilla (2006) identifies three approaches to integration utilized in interdisciplinary research, all of which involve decoding comparative disciplinary epistemologies: *conceptual bridging*, *comprehensiveness*, and *pragmatism*.

3. Science develops theories and laws, expressed in verbal, logical or mathematical forms, trough cycles of inductive and deductive processes. These will include data collection and observation, operationalization and investigation. Throughout history scientists and philosophers have defined disciplines in different ways. The nature of matter, living or nonliving, human or non-human, might contribute to define the boundaries of disciplines. The ways in which we sense and perceive, in qualitative and quantitative ways, are also contributing to define these boundaries. Measures, devices able to extend our sensory/perceptive capacity, algorithms, metaphors and models, might further contribute to change ways in which we can "cut" reality along different realms. What the ultimate real, *Das Ding an-Sich*, might be beyond our conventions, can be a matter for metaphysics and spirituality. Academia and research funding, with its social and financial constraints, will also contribute to shaping and reshaping disciplines. Then, disciplines might be defined as soft or hard depending from the amount of mathematics and statistics involved in studies and practice. It is possible that a study of the key role of metaphor in science and knowledge might also allow a better understanding of the interdisciplinary method (Orsucci, 1998, 2002, 2008). More recently, metaphors for describing knowledge have shifted from linear or hierarchical structures to networks, webs, textures in dynamic interaction. Welch (2009) links interdisciplinarity to a paradigm shift in the way we consider knowledge. Once described as a foundation or linear structure, knowledge today is depicted as a rhizome, a network or a web with multiple nodes of connection,

and as a dynamical system. The metaphor of unity, with its accompanying values of universality and certainty, has been replaced by metaphors of plurality and relationality, in a complex world. Images of boundary crossing, and cross-fertilization are superseding images of disciplinary depth and compartmentalization. Isolated modes of work are being supplanted by team working, and alliances. And, older values of competence, and expertise are being reformulated as partnership and negotiation. (Klein, 2004, 2010).

4. The US National Academy of Sciences (2005 CFR) definition is that "Interdisciplinary research is a mode of research in which a scientist or a team of scientists integrates information, data, techniques, tools, perspectives, concepts and/or theories, from two or more disciplines or bodies of specialized knowledge, with the objective to advance fundamental understanding or to solve problems whose solutions are beyond the scope of a single discipline or area of research practice." There might be different gradations of interbreeding or integration between disciplines, depending form different scholars. For example, Menken & Keestra (2016) propose three grades:

a. *Multidisciplinary*, some complementarity without integration and separate results;
b. *Interdisciplinarity*, with deeper integration and common results;
c. *Transdisciplinary*, including non-academic knowledge, with integrated results.

The design of and interdisciplinary study includes the implicit or explicit design of a new framework of patterns and algorithms shared throughout different disciplines. Potentially, there is a new hybrid structure that might emerge from old separated ones. "Seen as a whole, that larger set of variables and relationships can be fruitfully thought of as a complex system" (Newell, Wentworth, & Sebberson, 2001). He proposed that: "In particular, we can better understand and carry out interdisciplinary integration if we recognize we are attempting to identify and make sense out of the self-organizing pattern of a phenomenon modeled by a particular complex system," Newell's formulation of the theoretical framework for interdisciplinary studies is potentially fruitful. However, he doesn't take all the logical conclusions from its premises. A complex systems approach should imply that there are new patterns, structures and algorithms which can be unveiled by every interdisciplinary study. The degree of determinism or indeterminacy might vary, depending from the complexity of the field and the attitudes of the scholar or scientist. In any case, there might be a new emergence in waiting.

5. Interdisciplinarity has become a widespread mantra for research, now accompanied by a growing body of publications. The evaluation of these studies, however, remains one of the least-understood aspects. Julie Klein (Klein, 2010) reviewed interdisciplinary and transdisciplinary research evaluation. She defined parallels between research performance and evaluation, presenting seven generic principles for evaluation. Interdisciplinary and transdisciplinary research performance and evaluation are both generative processes of harvesting, capitalizing, and leveraging multiple expertise. Individual standards must be calibrated, and tensions among different disciplinary, professional, and interdisciplinary approaches carefully managed in balancing acts that require operative knowledge and epistemological negotiation and compromise. New epistemic communities are established, and new cultures of evidence produced. The multidisciplinary–interdisciplinary–transdisciplinary research environment spans a wide range of contexts. Klein is proposing seven pragmatic principles providing a coherent framework for thinking about evaluation of interdisciplinary studies: (1) variability of goals; (2) variability of criteria and indicators; (3) leveraging of integration; (4) interaction of social and cognitive factors in collaboration; (5) management, leadership, and coaching; (6) iteration in a comprehensive and transparent system; and (7) effectiveness and impact (Cunningham & Fitzgerald, 1996).

6. A deconstructionist approach, potentially avoiding the evidence/evaluation challenge, was proposed by Jacques Derrida, Jacques Foucault and others. This perspective devises the epistemological stance of *différance*. This neologism, a newly created compound word, acknowledges the separation of subject from object, and the Heideggerian notion that beings stand out, they differ. While at the same time, following Husserl, *différance* situates the subject in a state of suspension, a deferral of judgment. This is a phenomenological *Epoché,* a bracketing position in which the subject decides to interact without superimposing intellectual conceptualizations. *Différance,* therefore is a kind of transitional state, a play of differences between activity and passivity (Derrida, 2001). The poles of objectivity/subjectivity do not, for Derrida, merely oscillate they dance with each other in a dynamic relationship which possesses nuanced polyrhythms. Foucault's conceptualizations of the relationships of power, culture, and knowledge are at their base a deep reexamination of epistemology. For Foucault, truth is not absolute, but rather an episteme within which our notions of truth are determined by a culture. Those governing its language, its schemes of perception, its exchanges, its techniques, its values, the hierarchy of its practices (Foucault, 1971). Thus, for

Foucault, epistemology becomes the metacognitive realization of the process of truth formation, rather than the establishment of Truth itself. This epistemological strategy embraces uncertainty as a necessary condition for truth.

7. However, to pragmatists, knowledge is a tool to be evaluated by its effectiveness and efficacy: it is never certain. At any time and place, knowledge is that which helps the most people achieve satisfaction of their needs, including the need for more knowledge (Cunningham & Fitzgerald, 1996). Pragmatism sought to minimize the reductionism which had paralyzed previous epistemological strategies by forming a strong link between knowledge and action. “Pragmatism offers a conception of reason that is practical rather than intellectual, expressed in intelligent doings rather than abstract sayings. Adaptability is its hallmark, rather than mastery of unchanging universal principles” (Brandom, 2002). However, rather than simply modeling the theoretical on the practical, the pragmatists synthesize both these notions as adaptive, dynamic interactions between organism and environment (p. 18). Pragmatism courts a kind of epistemological balance, critical of the reductionism of the Western philosophical tradition, while simultaneously avoiding the nihilism intimated by postmodernism, and therefore is quite in line with modern interdisciplinary approach to knowledge.

8. This approach has been generating a specific pedagogy. As Gibbons (1979) has proposed: “What, logically, happens when concepts and propositions from different disciplines are brought together in a synthesis?” (Gibbons, 1979). Herbart’s notion of *apperceptive mass* changed the way theorists conceptualized the sequencing of learning (Herbart, 1891). *Integration* as being the final adjustment of a changing organism, or the successful completion of its growth depending on the nature of the environmental input. This evolutionary concept was quickly adopted by psychology, neurology, and physiology to indicate the stability of a whole organism, or the successful completion of adaptation of an organism that had been temporarily displaced or disturbed. Around 1916, *Gestalt* psychology popularized the notion that all parts of a system or organism can only be defined or understood by their relation to the whole (Relan & Kimpston, 1991). Furthermore, organismic psychology (as Gestalt was called in the United States) promoted a school curriculum that reflected an interconnected, authentic, environment that presumably provided maximum relevance or meaning to the whole child. Integration was seen on the one hand to be a means (the interactions, adaptations, and influences of parts of a system on the whole) and on the other hand to be an end (the successful completion of the

growth of an organism) (Knudsen, 1937). The view of integration as a means is apparent in the vast body of research in cognition. During the 1960s, Piaget's constructivist psychology and Bruner's structural cognitivism influenced the development of many innovative courses (Gozzer, 1982). Knowledge was viewed as 'something becoming,' something to construct through active inquiry. Learning was not simply the accumulation of facts but was believed to induce the restructuring of the learner's cognitive structure or organization (Marzano, 1991). Knowledge was increasingly seen as a complex, interconnected system requiring new pedagogical methods for successful learning to take place. Situated cognition, thematic organizers, and concept mapping have been ways of developing more receptive and connected curricula for students. Many such pedagogical concepts have been fundamental in shaping current interdisciplinary and integrated models.

Table 1. Levels of integration (Mathison & Freeman, 1998)

- intradisciplinary discipline-field
  - enhances connections within disciplines
  - promotes success for all students.
- cross-disciplinary correlated
  - coordinated themes/content across separate subjects
  - emphasis of certain skills across disciplines.
- interdisciplinary
  - processes, concepts, skills, or elements of two or more disciplines together
  - common themes or modes of inquiry form interdisciplinary connections
  - inquiry skills and discipline content are enhanced.
- integrated
  - disciplines lost in global perspective
  - theme or issue oriented
  - inquiry oriented.
- integrative
  - disciplines lost in global perspective
  - student/teacher negotiated themes and issues directed
  - inquiry oriented.

9. The view of integration as an end is associated with the growth in a child-centered curriculum that takes into account the whole child, including

physical, emotional, social, and cognitive needs. In holistic approaches "knowledge is perceived within experience and cannot be separated from the personal meaning given to it by the individual." Progressive educators like Dewey, an early proponent of an integrated curriculum, saw curriculum as a means to developing the critical attitudes in students that would enable them to participate as informed citizens in a democracy. Critical thinking goals, however, have either lost or gained popularity in direct relationship to socio-political events. Both brain response and higher-order thinking tasks were found to demand authentic, complex, multiple, and concrete problem-solving experiences (Marzano, 1991). This coupled with espoused workplace needs, which have advanced that all students need the skills to adapt, analyze, organize, and interpret fast-paced, multidimensional environments.

10. Disciplines are built on a compartmentalization determined by the need to gain thorough knowledge of the various aspects of each cognitive area. Criteria of reflection and study appropriate to each sector are determined, and there is a certain crystallization of the various fields of inquiry, defined by their characteristics of observability, method and application. What happens to the disciplines in interdisciplinarity? Are they linked, combined, restructured, transformed? However, most theorists see the disciplines as necessary stepping stones between current curricular approaches and truly integrated models of curriculum. There are many terms used in the literature interdisciplinary, core, fusion, integrated, cross-disciplinary, correlated, integrative, trans-disciplinary.

11. In summary then, an *interdisciplinary* approach combines two or more disciplines and keeps them distinct and in focus. It has clear objectives that include both critical-thinking skills and in-depth content and is typically teacher directed but may welcome student input. An *integrated* approach transcends disciplinary-bound knowledge in the exploration of a more unified and realistic view of knowledge. It is inquiry oriented and usually thematically based, and the themes and activities are teacher picked and directed. The goals are structured and include content, skills, and processes. Finally, an *integrative* approach starts with students' and teachers' concerns and ideas, transcends the disciplines in a search for coherence and meaning, and is built through daily negotiations and interactions. The goals are more affective and include such goals as personal relevance, collaboration, and citizenship skills. *Integrated* and *integrative* curricula require a complete restructuring or reconceptualization of what is meant by learning and teaching. Working within a framework of uncertainties is not easy. Especially in an integrative approach, where not only teachers but students are well enculturated in the

traditional authoritarian teaching-learning model, it is difficult to invest the time required to feel comfortable with and trust new roles, goals, and interactions. Jacobs infers that the biggest reason for the failure to establish an integrated curriculum is that teachers try too much too quickly and don't provide transitional time for themselves and their students (in Brandt, 1991). While an interdisciplinary model involves relatively little risk, an integrated or integrative approach involves a great deal of risk.

12. However, difficulties in the implementation of interdisciplinary or integrated approaches do not lie solely with lecturers. They report that their students were unable to overcome their dependence on disciplinary knowledge; had difficulty with unfamiliar open-ended tasks; and were either reluctant or unable to discuss information at deeper levels (Wicklein & Schell, 1995). Parents are also concerned their children did not learn enough facts, and that such approaches would lower their chances at getting into top Universities. In contrast to the tendencies of the Western epistemological tradition, complex systems are non-hierarchically structured. They obey multiple conflicting logics, employ both positive and negative feedback, reveal synergistic effects, and may have a chaotic element. To understand them, linear and reductionist thinking must be replaced by nonlinear thinking, pattern recognition, and analogy. Metaphors for describing knowledge have shifted from foundational and linear structures to networks, webs, and complex systems. Complexity is thus characterized as self-organizing, yet quasi-stable and dynamic (Klein, 1996, 2010). Newell contends that because interdisciplinarity inherently involves the negotiation of disciplinary perspectives, it is the nature of interdisciplinary inquiry to focus upon how the behavioral patterns of complex systems achieve coherence through the dynamic interaction of their constituent parts (Newell et al., 2001).

13. The idea of "A Theory of Interdisciplinarity" is by nature paradoxical and accepting this paradox to build a new approach on it. There have been many contenders, but none have achieved substantial traction (Klein & Newell, 1997). This is due, in part, to the ambivalence inherent in the interdisciplinary idea. Newell (2001) made one attempt in proposing complex systems theory as a model for an interdisciplinary research. Theory is tested by its systematicity and commensurability, rooted in close observation of phenomena and yielding generalizable conclusions about how nature works; yet the interdisciplinary approach to epistemology explicitly accepts that complex phenomena are at least partially indeterminate. Complexity, says Klein, asks more of theory than it can deliver. She argues that complex systems could aid interdisciplinary inquiry better in the guise of metaphor than in

theory. In "Interdisciplinary Thought," Ursula Hübenthal (1994) asserts that interdisciplinary collaboration is required because "these problems are much too complex to be judged appropriately, much less solved, merely with the subject-knowledge of a single discipline."

14. For example, interdisciplinary courses on phenomena modeled by complex systems promote desirable liberal education outcomes for students, and faculty development for their teachers. Interdisciplinary study prepares future professionals to confront the complex behaviors they will face on the job. It produces new knowledge by synthesizing insights from old knowledge about specific complex systems and by freeing scholars to ask new questions about them. It facilitates fundamental critique by viewing society or politics or knowledge as the dynamic product of a complex of interacting systemic forces. And by partially reorganizing the structure of the university around different categories of complex systems, it reduces the pressure for complete "coverage" of each discipline, thus eliminating an obstacle to downsizing. All seven motivations are consistent with the conception of interdisciplinarity presented in this paper. Clearly, the knowledge base in science is expanding too fast to ensure that students cover all aspects of scientific knowledge within the duration of a university course. The alternative is to offer students learning experiences that allow for conceptual exploration and acquisition of thinking skills needed for their future learning. 8

15. It is on this assumption that inspires learning environments for the development of metacognitive skills. Meta-cognitive knowledge refers to what a learner understands and believes about a subject matter or a task, and the judgments s/he makes in allocating cognitive resources as a result of that knowledge. Metacognitive control refers to the approaches and strategies a learner devises to achieve specific learning goals and the degree to which the learner organizes, monitors, and modifies those operations to ensure that learning is effective. Many students have rather primitive theories of learning and the demonstrate an epistemological perspective at a stage called basic dualism by (Kitchner, 1983). This stage is characterized by passivity and dependence on authority to hand down the truth and dictate what is right or wrong. In contrast, expert problem solvers demonstrate advanced skills and are able to operate independently to plan, monitor and control their learning.

16. Modern educational research affirms pedagogies and instructional approaches that emphasize the interaction of cognitive, metacognitive and affective components of learning. If educators only emphasize content and discrete skills, students may not develop the deep learning approaches that enable transfer of skills and knowledge to real world contexts. Metacognitive

skills are often distinguished from metacognitive knowledge (Hofer, 2001). The latter concept refers to the declarative knowledge one has about the interplay between personal characteristics, task characteristics, and available strategies in a learning situation (Flavell, 1999). Metacognitive skills, on the other hand, concern the procedural knowledge that is required for the personal characteristics, task characteristics, and available strategies in a learning situation (Flavell, 1999). Metacognitive skills, on the other hand, concern the procedural knowledge that is required for the actual regulation of and control over one's learning activities (Kuhn, 2000). Task analysis, planning, monitoring, checking, and reflection are manifestations of such skills. The question is whether metacognition can be reduced to cognition. Indeed, follow-up studies showed that metacognition was only partially independent of intelligence. Flavell (1999) related the concept of metacognition to Piaget's developmental stage of formal- operational thinking (Inhelder & Piaget, 1958).

17. There might be more to explore in a possible theory of interdisciplinary practice, areas of research and theoretical studies where similar tools and methodologies are being used in different disciplines. This kind of science practice has been producing explicit and implicit interdisciplinarity since ancient times. More recently it has reached new levels of refinement. It is also compounded by the travelling of some groups of scholars through different disciplines. Let's have a look at some modern examples of the second phenomenon which can help us to highlight more also of the first one. Mitchell Jay Feigenbaum (born December 19, 1944) is a mathematical physicist whose pioneering studies in chaos theory led to the discovery of the Feigenbaum constants. In 1986, he was awarded the Wolf Prize in Physics "for his pioneering theoretical studies demonstrating the universal character of non-linear systems, which has made possible the systematic study of chaos." In 1975, Dr. Feigenbaum, using the small HP-65 calculator he had been issued, discovered that the ratio of the difference between the values at which such successive period-doubling bifurcations occur tends to a constant of around 4.6692... He was able to provide a mathematical proof of that fact, and he then showed that the same behavior, with the same mathematical constant, would occur within a wide class of mathematical functions, prior to the onset of chaos. For the first time, this universal result enabled mathematicians to take their first steps to unraveling the apparently intractable "random" behavior of chaotic systems. This "ratio of convergence" is now known as the first Feigenbaum constant. The logistic map is a prominent example of the mappings that Feigenbaum studied in his

noted 1978 article: Quantitative Universality for a Class of Nonlinear Transformations (Feigenbaum, 1978).

18. Feigenbaum's other contributions include important new fractal methods in cartography, starting when he was hired by Hammond to develop techniques to allow computers to assist in drawing maps. Using fractal geometry to describe natural forms such as coastlines, mathematical physicist Feigenbaum developed software capable of reconfiguring coastlines, borders, and mountain ranges to fit a multitude of map scales and projections (Feigenbaum, 1994). In another practical application of his work, he founded *Numerix* with Michael Goodkin in 1996. The company's initial product was a software algorithm that dramatically reduced the time required for Monte Carlo pricing of exotic financial derivatives and structured products. *Numerix* remains one of the leading software providers to financial markets. Its website declares: "*Numerix* next generation technology solutions help Banks manage the complexities of the changing capital markets landscape, effectively manage risk and build a competitive edge." Feigenbaum is just one of the most prominent examples of researchers jumping with nonchalance the boundaries between different disciplines. Physicists have been moving to economy and finance in massive migrations since new models and investing techniques developed in the last years. Migrations didn't involve only scholars. There has been also the spreading of models and methods. Some methodology and modelling have been produced within one discipline, but scholars moved to apply to in other neighboring or more distant areas. Network theory, for example, started in mathematics, was further developed by sociologists and then exploited and widely implemented in computer science. There are many other possible examples in the direction of time series analysis and statistics: Markov chains, Recurrence Quantification Analysis, principal components analysis, cellular automata and network theory. etc.

19. The main driver in this new grounded approach to multidisciplinary studies has been research and applications to complex problems and phenomena. The widespread availability of hardware and software with exponentially increased capacity has certainly helped to deal with these areas previously considered beyond our capability. Complex Adaptive Systems (CAS) or complex systems are characterized by the interactions between their numerous elements. The word 'complex' comes from the Latin *plexus* which means entwined. In other words, it is difficult to correlate global properties of complex systems with the properties of the individual constituent components. This is primarily because the interactions between these individual elements partly determine the future states of the system. If these interactions are not

included in the developed models, the models would not be an accurate reflection of the modelled phenomenon. While numerous techniques and frameworks for modeling complex systems have previously been devised, clearly one of the most explicit and intuitive methodology is the modeling of interactions using networks (Niazi & Hussain, 2012). Networks consist of nodes or vertices, which can be used to represent elements, and links or edges, which usually represent interactions or relations between the elements. In this context, networks represent the structure of complex systems; how elements interact. However, networks can also be used to represent the dynamics or function of complex systems, e.g., considering nodes as states and links as transitions. Thus, the same analysis can be applied to the structure and the function of networks.

20. Understanding the relationship between structure and function is one of the major open questions across sciences, which can also be posed using networks: how do changes in the structural network affect the state network? For example, what will be the effect of knocking out a gene in the behavior of a cell? Several systems change their structure over time, and their properties can be modelled with temporal networks. Likewise, there are several instances when the structural changes are triggered by the state of the network, as has been studied in adaptive networks. With not much more than a decade of network research, there are already numerous applications of networks in diverse areas, such as epidemiology, human mobility, social networks, artificial life, life sciences, theory of computation, and engineering, just to mention a few (Barabasi & Frangos, 2003; Newman, Barabasi, & Watts, 2011).

21. The impact of complexity science on multidisciplinary collaborations leads a general redesign of epistemology. We assist to the emergence of a new meta-level of scientific elaboration which strengthens the role of mathematical modelling and statistical analysis as methodologies crossing throughout various fields and necessary for scientific evidence in multiple disciplines. This movement shows that vast areas of the humanities are now accessible to formal quantitative and qualitative methods. A recent and strong example is represented by the area of social media (traditional and internet based) where mostly network based methodologies and big data approaches are now mainstream. This means that there are new ways for recognizing, analyzing and modelling emerging algorithms and patterns across different disciplines. The full epistemological maturity of this new approach is still to be reached but, perhaps, not too far away. As Hooker (2011) highlights, science has discovered the phenomenal richness and explanatory power of complex

systems. However, a general model of the complex organization of dynamical processes is not yet developed, possibly because a "theory of everything" is not in the nature of scientific methods. So, what is considered a "lack of a general foundation" is just inherent to the scientific method in general. At the same time, we can see that "complex systems methodology and philosophy" can provide a meta level of abstraction which can subsume and remold disciplinary domains and boundaries.

22. Therefore, we can return to the classic paper by Warren Weaver on science and complexity (1948 in Weaver, 1991) to consider how realistic and visionary at the same time it was. He divided his reflections in three parts. In the first part he was summing up that "physical science before 1900 was largely concerned with two-variable *problems of simplicity*; whereas the life sciences, in which these problems of simplicity are not so often significant, had not yet become highly quantitative or analytical in character." *Problems of disorganized complexity* became paradoxically more tractable since the advent of reliable probability theory and statistical mechanics. This left as most difficult a large region in the middle which he called of *organized complexity*: "They are all problems which involve dealing simultaneously with a sizable number of factors which are interrelated into an organic whole." (Weaver, 1948). A wide range of similar problems in the biological, medical, psychological, economic, and political sciences- are just too complicated to yield to the old nineteenth-century techniques which were so dramatically successful on two-, three-, or four-variable problems of simplicity. These new problems, moreover, cannot be handled with the statistical techniques so effective in describing average behavior in problems of disorganized complexity. He then makes two examples related to his recent wartime experience which are so immediately relevant for this inquiry. He first mentioned that the development of modern computers with their combination of flexibility, capacity and speed would have such an impact in future science. The second example is that the wartime advances in science were related to the implementation of the *mixed team approach* of operations analysis. These groups were first proposed by British teams, notably at Bletchley Park, but soon afterwards adopted also by the Americans. Under the pressure of war, these mixed teams pooled their resources and focused all their different insights on the common problems. It was found, in spite of the modern tendencies toward intense scientific specialization, that "members of such diverse groups could work together and could form a unit which was much greater than the mere sum of its parts." It was shown that these groups could tackle certain problems of organized complexity and get useful answers.

Therefore, they could challenge at the same time boundaries between disciplines and boundaries of what was considered as possible science in dealing with difficult and complex problems. Problem solving, team working, communication and critical thinking are still crucial factors for the advancement of science and are on top of the skills agenda in preparing students for future challenges in science, workplaces and everyday life. Interdisciplinary knowledge is already progressing towards an integrative understanding of dynamical algorithms and patterns.

References

Barabasi, A. L., & Frangos, J. (2003). *Linked: The New Science of Networks*. New York: Perseus Books.

Brandom, R. (2002). Explanatory vs. expressive deflationism about truth. In R. Schantz ed. *What Is Truth*? Berlin: De Gruyter.

Cunningham, J. W., & Fitzgerald, J. (1996). Epistemology and reading. *Reading Research Quarterly*, 31(1), 36-60.

Derrida, J. (2001). *Writing and difference*. London: Routledge.

Feigenbaum, M. J. (1978). Quantitative universality for a class of nonlinear transformations. *Journal of Statistical Physics*, 19(1), 25-52.

Feigenbaum, M. J. (1994). Riemann maps and world maps. In *Trends and perspectives in applied mathematics* (pp. 55-71). Berlin: Springer.

Flavell, J. H. (1999). Cognitive development: Children's knowledge about the mind. *Annual Review of Psychology*, 50(1), 21-45.

Foucault, M. (1971). *The order of things an archaeology of the human sciences* (Vol. 1st American ed.). New York: Pantheon Books.

Gibbons, J. A. (1979). Curriculum integration. *Curriculum Inquiry*, 9(4), 321-332.

Gozzer, G. (1982). Interdisciplinarity: a concept still unclear. *Prospects*, 12(3), 281-292.

Herbart, J. F. (1891). *A text-book in psychology: An attempt to found the science of psychology on experience, metaphysics, and mathematics* (Vol. 18). D. Appleton.

Hofer, B. K. (2001). Personal epistemology research: Implications for learning and teaching. *Educational Psychology Review*, 13(4), 353-383.

Hooker, C. (2011). Introduction to philosophy of complex systems: A. *Philosophy of Complex Systems*, 10(3).

Inhelder, B., & Piaget, J. (1958). The growth oflogical thinking. *From Childhood to Adolescence*. 13.

Kitchner, K. S. (1983). Cognition, metacognition, and epistemic cognition. *Human Development*, 26(4), 222-232.

Klein, J. T. (1996). *Crossing boundaries: Knowledge, disciplinarities, and interdisciplinarities*. University of Virginia Press.

Klein, J. T. (2010). A taxonomy of interdisciplinarity. *The Oxford Handbook of Interdisciplinarity*, 15, 15-30.

Klein, J. T., & Newell, W. H. (1997). Advancing interdisciplinary studies. *Handbook of the Undergraduate Curriculum: A Comprehensive Guide to Purposes, Structures, Practices, and Change*, 393-415.

Knudsen, C. W. (1937). What do educators mean by "integration." *Harvard Educational Review*, 7(1), 15-26.

Kuhn, D. (2000). Metacognitive development. *Current Directions in Psychological Science*, 9(5), 178-181.

Mansilla, V. B. (2006). Assessing expert interdisciplinary work at the frontier: an empirical exploration. *Research Evaluation*, 15(1), 17-29.

Marzano, R. J. (1991). Fostering thinking across the curriculum through knowledge restructuring. *Journal of Reading*, 34(7), 518-525.

Mathison, S., & Freeman, M. (1998). The Logic of Interdisciplinary Studies. *Report Series* 2.33.

Menken, S., & Keestra, M. (2016). *An introduction to interdisciplinary research: theory and practice*. Amsterdam University Press.

Newell, W. H. (1998). *Interdisciplinarity: Essays from the literature*. College Board.

Newell, W. H., Wentworth, J., & Sebberson, D. (2001). A theory of interdisciplinary studies. *Issues in Interdisciplinary Studies*.

Newman, M., Barabasi, A.-L., & Watts, D. J. (2011). *The structure and dynamics of networks* (Vol. 19). Princeton University Press.

Niazi, M. A., & Hussain, A. (2012). *Cognitive agent-based computing-I: a unified framework for modeling complex adaptive systems using agent-based & complex network-based methods*. Berlin: Springer. 14.

Orsucci, F. (1998). *The Complex Matters of the Mind.* River Edge, NJ; World Scientific.

Orsucci, F. (2002). *Changing Mind Transitions in Natural and Artificial Environments.* River Edge, NJ: World Scientific.

Orsucci, F. (2012). *Complexity Science, Living Systems, and Reflexing Interfaces.* New York: IGI International.

Popper, K. R. (1968). Epistemology without a knowing subject. In *Studies in Logic and the Foundations of Mathematics* (Vol. 52, pp. 333-373). London: Elsevier.

Popper, K. R. (1974). Scientific reduction and the essential incompleteness of all science. In *Studies in the Philosophy of Biology* (pp. 259-284). Berlin: Springer.

Relan, A., & Kimpston, R. (1991). Curriculum Integration: A Critical Analysis of Practical and Conceptual Issues. *Proceedings, Annual Meeting of the American Educational Research Association* (Chicago, IL, April 3-7, 1991)

Weaver, W. (1991). Science and complexity. In *Facets of Systems Science* (pp. 449-456). Berlin: Springer.

Welch IV, J. L. (2009). *Interdisciplinarity and the history of ideas*. The University of Texas at Dallas.

Wicklein, R. C., & Schell, J. W. (1995). Case studies of multidisciplinary approaches to integrating mathematics, science and technology education. *Journal of Technology Education*, 6(2), 59-76.

Chapter 2

Indirect Biological Measures of Consciousness from Field Studies of Brains as Dynamical Systems*

Walter J. Freeman†
Department of Molecular and Cell Biology, University of California at Berkeley, Berkeley, CA, USA

Abstract

Consciousness fully supervenes when the 1.5 kg mass of protoplasm in the head directs the body into material and social environments and engages in reciprocity. While consciousness is not susceptible to direct measurement, a limited form exercised in animals and pre-lingual children can be measured indirectly with biological assays of arousal, intention and attention. In this essay consciousness is viewed as operating simultaneously in a field at all levels ranging from subatomic to social. The relations and transpositions between levels require sophisticated mathematical treatments that are largely still to be devised.

In anticipation of those developments the available experimental data are reviewed concerning the state variables in several levels that collectively constitute the substrate of biological consciousness. The basic metaphors are described that represent the neural machinery of transposition in consciousness. The processes are sketched by which spatiotemporal neural activity patterns emerge as fields that may represent the contents of consciousness.

* This article was originally published in Chaos and Complexity Letters, volume 4 number 3 (2010).

† Corresponding Author's E-mail: drwjfiii@berkeley.edu.

In: Neuroscience and Technology Transform the Educational Ecosystem
Editors: Franco F. Orsucci and Nicoletta Sala
ISBN: 979-8-88697-157-6

The results of dynamical analysis are discussed in terms serving to distinguish between the neural point processes dictated by the neuron doctrine vs. continuously variable neural fields generated by neural masses in cortex.

Keywords: action-perception cycle, arousal, attention, attractor landscape, consciousness, criticality, electroencephalogram (EEG), fields, intention, phase transition, wave packet

1. Introduction

Dynamical systems are collections of entities that organize themselves into continually changing groups by exchanging matter and energy. Examples range in scale from molecules of air and water creating hurricanes to citizens creating committees. Dynamical brain systems likewise range from quantum excitation of receptors to molecules that organize into DNA, proteins and membranes to people collectively creating tribes and teams. Entities that support consciousness operate simultaneously as a seamless whole across the entire range. Owing to their diversity the scientific study of these entities requires measurement at different scales of time and space. Each study has its own experimental paradigm and theory by which to relate brain structures and functions to consciousness through behaviors. Physiologists record trains of action potentials of axons and local field potentials (LFP) of dendrites in relation to perceptions reported by subjects of objects and people; they explain their findings with help from anatomists using Golgi stains to reveal neurons in networks and sophisticated histochemical techniques that reveal large-scale neural organization. Neurochemists and pharmacologists collaborate with electron microscopists and geneticists to analyze the ultrastructures of membranes, vesicles and DNA in order to understand the hereditary and experiential determinants of memory. Psychologists and engineers correlate behaviors with noninvasive brain images of regional variations in blood flow, the concentrations of chemicals (glucose, oxygen, hemoglobin, radiolabeled neurotransmitters), magnetic fields (magnetoencephalogram, (MEG) and electric fields (electroencephalogram, EEG) in order to localize cortical and nuclear modules that are coactive with intentional behaviors. Sociologists use clinical observations on subjects with neurogenetic or drug-induced disorders of brain functions to explain maladaptive behaviors and altered states. Every reflex and intentional act and thought is based in exchanges of matter and energy through neural activity at every scale.

Our need to comprehend the mind-boggling diversity of forms and scales of matter and energy and their rates of change imposes the requirement for a universal language with which to describe relationships among them. That language is mathematics. In research by my groups over the past half century we have constructed one such language, a hierarchical system of differential equations called Katchalsky models ("K-sets") which are designed and parameterized using anatomical, pharmacological, and physiological data, and which serve to simulate and explain virtually all of our experimental observations on brain activity in relation to behavior (Freeman, 1975, 2000; Kozma and Freeman, 2001; Principe et al., 2001; Kozma, Freeman and Erdí, 2003). This is not to say that the language of brains is mathematics. The leading 20th century mathematician John von Neumann wrote: "…the mathematical or logical language truly used by the central nervous system is characterized by less logical and arithmetical depth than what we are normally used to. …We require exquisite numerical precision over many logical steps to achieve what brains accomplish in very few short steps. ... Whatever the system is, it cannot fail to differ considerably from what we consciously and explicitly consider as mathematics (1958, pp. 80-81)". Rather, mathematics in many forms provides tools that investigators use to measure and represent the relations of brain functions to behavior, cognition, and consciousness.

Although differential equations form the core of my inferences, like other skeletons they are best relegated to the closets of appendices and monographs. My aim in this essay is to describe in words my view of brain dynamics with the particular intent of explaining some properties that are inferred for consciousness. My Introduction and Section 2 list the major levels of brain function in consciousness and give examples of the state variables at each level, representing the *substances* of consciousness and leading to discussion of the relations and transpositions of measurements across levels. Section 3 contrasts descriptions of brain operations on the one hand in terms of information carried by action potentials and on the other hand in terms of knowledge fragments expressed in fields of neural activity that are manifested in epiphenomenal electric and magnetic field potentials (EEG and MEG), which support discussion and comparison of the reflex arc and the action-perception cycle representing basic neural *machineries* of consciousness. Section 4 takes up the problems posed by intentional action and proposed solutions in terms of self-stabilizing background activity and the formation, transmission, and integration of self-organized spatiotemporal patterns of goal-directed brain activity that may represent the *contents* of consciousness. Section 5 summarizes implications of dynamics for further specific *properties* of consciousness.

There are severe constraints on what can be achieved with this neurodynamical approach to consciousness. There is no universally accepted definition of consciousness or agreement on variant types, levels and altered states. There is no physiological measure or index of consciousness. The only test available is to ask a subject: "Are you conscious now, and do you remember being so in the past?" Animal subjects that provide functional data cannot pass this test, and no one has yet succeeded in proving precise neural correlates in humans of verbal or otherwise symbolic reports of self-referential experiences. Therefore my remarks on properties of consciousness refer to a state that I conceive to exist in animals and small children before they can talk. I leave the 'hard problem' (Chalmers, 1996) to philosophers and limit my comments to some not-too-surprising biological properties that I conceive as emergent from modeling brain dynamics, namely that consciousness arises in a very small and intermittent fraction of the variance from the enormous groundswell of widely distributed background brain activity in intentional states; that the contents form entirely by endogenous construction of macroscopic patterns ultimately from microscopic cellular input and not by import of forms through the senses; that the contents are in fields that are globally distributed over each hemisphere though neither uniformly, homogeneously, nor reproducibly; that the stream of consciousness is cinematographic rather than continuous, with multiple frames in coalescing rivulets; that its action in respect to contents is judgmental rather than enactive, so that its prime role is not to make decisions but to delay and defer action and thereby minimize premature commitment of limited resources. This aspect is couched in the adage: "stop and think before acting".

There remains the question whether it might be possible to put forward in the biological context an acceptable definition of consciousness that incorporates the subjective, experiential property of consciousness. While for many philosophers consciousness poses an enigma and a mystery (Searle, 1995), there is no doubt about the immediacy and primacy of the experience, which strongly resembles our experience of diverse kinds of force and energy, whether inertial, gravitational, electric, thermal, etc. We can only indirectly experience forces by observing their effects on persons and objects that are accessible to our sensory and perceptual neural mechanisms. We measure each kind of force by its effects on objects in motion. In this essay I pursue this analogy and come to the conclusion that consciousness is not merely 'like' a force; it *is* a field of force that can be understood in the same ways that we understand all other fields of force (and energy) within which we, through our bodies, are immersed, and which we, through our bodies, comprehend in accordance with the known laws of physics.

2. The Flow of Activity through Dynamical Systems and Its Description as Information

The study of brain activity at every scale must include measurements of intentional and voluntary behaviors, if the tables, graphs and illustrations that display the properties of molecules, organelles, neural networks, populations, modules, and large-scale brain systems are to be meaningful. The difficulties of that search for meaning are reflected in the conflicts and uncertainties that are encountered in the search for the neural correlates of consciousness. There are wide explanatory gaps between observations of brain activity and verbal reports of phenomenological experiences and intended or voluntary actions. Dynamical systems theory may help to bridge those gaps and demonstrate the relevance of the pulse trains from microelectrodes and the brain patches from functional magnetic resonance imaging (fMRI) to the concerns of psychiatrists, philosophers, theologians, jurisprudents, politicians, estheticians and advertisers. In order to make the bridges neurodynamicists must show how small-scale entities self-organize through forming large-scale entities and transforming and modulating themselves in the circular process. The requisite interactions, variously termed circular causality or feedback whether recurrent or reentrant, occur through serial stages across synaptic connections and non-synaptic channels (Freeman, 2005b) that form chains and both forward and feedback loops. These multi-level dynamic interrelations are schematized by the topological networks of K-sets (Freeman, 1975; Kozma, Freeman and Erdi, 2003).

A well-understood example of serial transformations across forms and scales is provided by the nerve-muscle preparation. The firing rates of axons (cellular events in electrochemical and magnetic energy) are related to the rates of transmitter release at synapses (molecular events in chemical energy), and these are related to the amplitudes of membrane and metabolic potentials of muscle cells (organelle events) and to the strengths of muscular contractions (system events in mechanical energy). A more sophisticated preparation is provided by a sensory system in an anesthetized subject. A stimulus to a receptor activates serially a molecular deformation, a cascading biochemical reaction, a generator potential, a train of action potentials transmitted to the brain, a release of packets of a chemical transmitter, and an activation of synaptic potentials in secondary neurons at a relay in a pathway to cortex. A tertiary neuron, usually thalamic, drives cortical neurons by further chains of chemoelectric transformations, culminating in frontal and parietal activity patterns that ultimately have social significance.

In an awake subject engaged with the environment those driven cortical neurons, even before stimulation, are already self-organized and active through intracortical and extracortical feedback loops. Small numbers of neurons form networks; tens of thousands of neurons form populations; hundreds of millions form modules. The excitatory interactions among neurons support the formation of continually evolving spatial patterns of cortical activity. The inhibitory interactions sharpen and bound those patterns. The interactions among excitatory and inhibitory neurons generate oscillations loosely called brain waves. Spatiotemporal patterns emerge of axonal, synaptic, and dendritic activity in the forms of trains of action potentials, local field potentials (LFP, EEG, MEG), event-related potentials (ERP), and varying rates of dissipation of metabolic energy that demand increased blood flow, from which enhanced activity is deduced. Focused responding to stimuli that subjects have learned to discriminate is accompanied by excitation of cortical neurons singly (feature detectors, cardinal cells, synfire chains, Hebbian networks), in populations (oscillatory brain waves with high vs. low amplitude modulations), and in modules (increases in regional blood flow to meet neural metabolic requirements).

At this point we encounter a major epistemological problem. The patterns of neural activity, which we correlate with conditioned stimuli and behaviors, feed on diverse forms of energy. Observers measure the various energy forms and express their quantities in numbers. The diversity of forms and scales is surmounted by treating the patterns in the numbers as information. The sequential transformations of the information are described with equations from information theory, and the measured spatial patterns, temporal oscillations and transformations are simulated by solving the equations. These numerical sequences and models provide the backbone of our knowledge about brain functions underlying consciousness. The equations serve to make models of "information processing", which has become not only a prime method of discovery but also the leading metaphor for describing brain functions in contemporary neuroscience.

It is important to recognize, as in the case of mathematics, that the information is in the dynamic systems models and not in the brain activity that it models. The reason is that brains create, store, retrieve and utilize knowledge from experience, but the knowledge of each subject is unique to that subject, and it is highly resistant to description in terms of information (Bartlett, 1932; Lucky, 1989). Some of the information that investigators define and deliver to sense organs is certainly incorporated into the knowledge of the subject, but the identity of the information is not preserved or measured, as it can be in a model of the perceptual process. When the model is confused with what it represents, investigators encounter the symbol grounding problem (Harnad, 1999), which has plagued artificial intelligence for half a century: how is a representation in the brain connected with what it represents in the world? For this reason representational and information-processing models fail, and alternative approaches must be explored. The search for alternatives is done by stepping back to broaden one's point of view.

3. Comparison of the Reflex Arc and the Action-Perception Cycle

An experimental subject engaged with the environment in a task forms a dynamical system in the form of a circular process that incorporates both subject and object at all levels simultaneously from subatomic to social (Pribram, 1991; Jibu et al., 1996; Chapline, 1999). The dynamics is analyzed by entering the cycle at either of two starting points: the reflex arc begins outside the brain, and the action-perception cycle begins inside the brain. Each conception has advantages and limitations, so they are complementary. Each stems from a different paradigm, so they are incompatible. The reflex arc is conceived by neuroscientists in Newtonian terms of point-to-point transmission of intensive trains of action potentials from identified neurons having high impact on selected target neurons at the synapses. The oscillations manifesting the impacts have fixed frequencies at zero phase lag (Engel et al., 1991; Schillen and König, 1994; Melloni et al., 2007), which is compatible only with stationarity and instantaneous action-at-a-distance. As with point mass, the energy (firing rate) is positive-valued. The intensities index the probability that a given signal is present (Barlow, 1972). Contrastingly the action-perception arc is conceived by neuroscientists in terms of Maxwellian fields (Köhler, 1940; Pribram, 1991; John, 2001; Tononi and Edelman, 2000) of low-density activity that is based in the effectively continuous distributions of synaptic energy in populations with billions of synapses/mm^3 (Freeman, 1975, 2000). The field energy is everywhere, not just at the axon terminals as postulated in a discrete network. Transmission in the establishment of co-active domains is not instantaneous action-at-a-distance but involves propagation delays, which are most clearly seen in the radially symmetric spatial patterns of phase having the form of right cones (Figure 1) that characterize the oscillations of wave packets ("phase cones", Freeman, 2004). The energy values that characterize the spatial patterns are bivalent; low or zero values are just as important as high values for identification and classification, because patterns require black and gray as well as white.

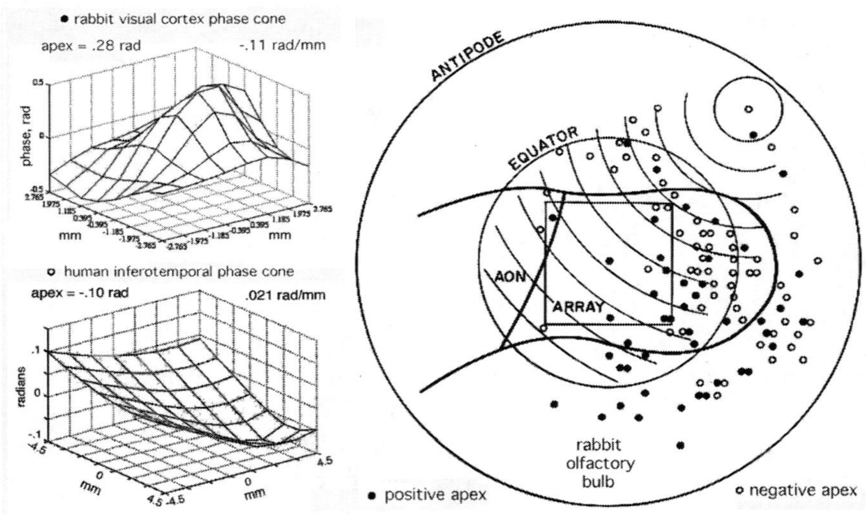

Figure 1. *Left:* examples of phase cones from neocortical electrocorticogram (ECoG, which is EEG recorded directly from cortical surfaces) of human (Freeman et al., 2006) and rabbit (Freeman, 2004b). *Right*: outline of rabbit bulb with square array superimposed on the opened spherical surface. The arcs show a representative phase cone; the dark symbols • show the locations of positive apices ("explosion"); the light symbols ° show negative apices ("implosion") (Freeman and Baird, 1987). The phase gradients of phase cones are measured in radians/mm. Biologically the gradients are determined by the ratio of the frequency of the shared oscillation in radians/s to the conduction velocities of axons running parallel to the cortical surface in m/s. The phase patterns and the random variation in sign at the apex from each frame to the next can only be explained by field theory. From Freeman (2007).

This contrast in 21st century neuroscience resembles that in 19th century physics between Newtonian interpretations of electric and magnetic forces in terms of point charges *vs.* the fields of Faraday and Maxwell (Barrett, 2000, 2001; Arianrhod, 2005). Then and now the contrasting views are polar opposites; neither view can be used to critique the other, because the divergence begins with the design of the experiments that are needed to collect the raw data to test them (Kuhn, 1962).

The activity in the reflex arc is initiated by an investigator who selects a sensory modality and gives a stimulus with information content that is measured in its features and intensities. The electrochemical responses to the stimulus are measured serially in the sensory receptors, the ascending pathways to cortex, and the hierarchy of cortical networks and modules, for example, V1>V2>V3>V4. The investigator selects rapidly firing neurons that provide high-density information in small numbers of neurons. The measurements provide the basis for seeking the information that was delivered in the stimulus and calculating the transformations by which that information flows through the brain. The transformations support deductions on how the information is processed, extracted, stored in memory, retrieved, compared with new information, and used to make decisions, select responses, and implement them by movements of the body into the environment, thereby closing the cycle from which the stimulus came. The success of the models is evaluated by calculating deviations between the measured observations and the simulations derived by solving the equations. This approach is well suited for the design, execution and interpretation of experiments in stimulus-response determinism using the behaviorist tools of schedules of reinforcement (Ferster and Skinner, 1957). However, the reflex arc cannot describe brain processes of intending goals, planning actions, predicting sensory consequences, attending to input, and creating knowledge by generalizing and abstracting, because as already stated those processes are knowledge-based, not information-based. From a broader perspective the goal of modeling reflex behavior is in the mind of the investigator: to control the subjects' behaviors by the systematic use of reward and punishment. The intentional cycle, of which the conventional reflex arc is one part, begins with the intention of the investigator, extends through the experimental subject, and is closed with the evaluation by the investigator of the conditioned response to the conditioned stimulus, as that stimulus is conceived by the investigator and not as it is perceived by the subject. Hence the reflex model can be subsumed into the action-perception model, but not the reverse.

The activity in the action-perception cycle of Piaget (1930) and Merleau-Ponty (1942) begins with a macroscopic state in the brain that embodies a goal. It emerges in the brain by extrapolation from recent and current input that is embedded in the context of the knowledge base. This predictive state implicitly contains nested mesoscopic activity patterns, which are constructed in corticostriatal and corticocerebellar modules (Houk, 2005), and which mediate the control of the body movements by the motor systems that the macroscopic state predicts may satisfy extant needs. The motor systems transmit to the brain stem and spinal cord the microscopic command patterns of action potentials that implement specific body movements of approach (e. g., grasping) or avoidance (e. g., flight). The descending action patterns include controls of the postural, autonomic and neuroendocrine back-ups for the expected action (commonly identified with expressions of emotions). The cortical modules also organize patterns called corollary discharges (Sperry, 1950), CODAM (Taylor, 2003), and efference copies (von Holst and Mittelstaedt, 1950) that are transmitted to the sensory systems. This process, also called preafference (Kay and Freeman, 1998), conveys to sensory cortices the expectations of the probable sensory consequences of the anticipated action. Phenomenologically the expectations may be experienced as states of desire, fear, lust, rage, etc. Biologically the expectations in sensory cortices have the form of selective sensitivities that are described as landscapes of chaotic attractors in brain state space (Viana Di Prisco and Freeman, 1985; Skarda and Freeman, 1987). Each attractor supports a dynamic memory embodied in a nerve cell assembly that has been shaped by synaptic changes under reinforcement and other forms of learning. Selection of an assembly leads to activation of an attractor and its stored memory, which is manifested in the emergence of a spatial pattern of amplitude modulation (AM) of a carrier wave in the gamma or beta frequency range. As noted in more detail in the next section, the AM patterns lack invariance with respect to conditioned stimuli (Barrie, Freeman and Lenhart, 1996; Ohl, Scheich and Freeman, 2001); they change with altered reinforcement contingencies or simply with the addition of new conditioned stimuli in serial conditioning (Freeman and Grajski, 1987; Freeman, 2005a). Therefore, they do not represent stimuli symbolically or otherwise; they express individual knowledge about the stimuli but well below the level of consciousness. Therefore the symbol grounding problem is not encountered.

A basin of attraction, metaphorically resembling a crater on the moon, surrounds each attractor. The basins form a landscape that the sensory cortex holds up to the world containing the set of predicted possible outcomes of an action into the world. Each possible outcome of an act of observation (such as an odor of food, a predator, a mate, the background, or a novel, unknown stimulus) leads by serial constructions in the forebrain to an appropriate follow-up behavior (approach, escape, orienting, etc.). All attractors are latent prior to an act of observation, upon which only one can be selected. Only one AM pattern can emerge as the outcome of the impact of the sensory volley on the expectant cortex. This outcome may appear to resemble the affordance of J. J. Gibson (1979), but it differs in the following respect. Gibson wrote: "... the affordance, being invariant, is always there to be perceived. An affordance is not bestowed upon an object by a need of an observer and his act of perceiving it. The object offers what it does because of what it is" (p. 139.) In other words the Gibsonian view holds that perceptual information is in the object and is transferred by resonances into the observer. Since there is no limit on the number of observers, each with individual resonances, the information content in the object is unbounded. Contrastingly in the proposed neurodynamic view the knowledge about the utilities of the object is in the attractor landscapes that are unique for each observer, not in the objects under observation.

A goal-oriented action predictably changes the relations of the senses to the environment, as when the eyes move and the visual fields appear to move oppositely. The barrages of sensory-evoked action potentials impact the sensory cortices, destabilize them, and activate their attractor landscapes by phase transitions. The sensory input to each sensory cortex in the several modalities selects one of the basins, and the dynamics converges to the attractor in the basin. The attractor governs the neural interactions that generate an oscillatory field of neural activity called a wave packet (Freeman, 1975). The mesoscopic wave packet differs from sensory-driven spike trains in two main respects. First, the domain of coherent oscillation in small mammals is very large, typically 15-30 mm in diameter (Freeman, 2004b), which includes and integrates ("binds") all subdivisions in each primary sensory area. Second, the information in the measurements of the AM pattern that serves for classification with respect to conditioned stimuli and responses is distributed and holographic; no one channel of EEG has more or less value than any other, whether the amplitude of oscillation is high, low or zero. Therefore, the same content of the wave packet is broadcast by action potentials of pyramidal cells simultaneously to all targets of the hierarchy of modules in the primary sensory areas, just as each fragment of a hologram contains the entire picture though at reduced resolution. The spatial AM patterns of the multiple sensory wave packets signal the same perceptual outcomes of the intentional action to all brain targets about the current status of the body with respect to the environment, signaling which of the expected outcomes has been selected in every modality but without the necessity for consciousness.

The convergence to an attractor in each cortex performs two operations: it abstracts the input, because convergence is independent of where in the basin of attraction the stimulus receptors happen to place the cortex, and it generalizes to a signal of the category to which a stimulus is assigned, because the attractor is based in the knowledge that has been accumulated by experience, not in the transient stimulus information. This point bears repetition. The stimulus information is unique, ephemeral, material and ultimately unknowable. For example, an odorant excites a specific subset of available receptors, but brains do not know or need to know which receptors. The outcome of convergence to an attractor is an AM pattern that expresses an abstract category that exists only in the brain. To be sure, the AM pattern is material, evanescent, never twice identical but sufficiently reproducible to be correctly classified on repetition over trials. This distinction in essence is that between matter and mind.

The firing of receptors can properly be said to represent a sensory event to the brain, where the action potentials from sensory relays select an attractor that activates a fragment of knowledge. The AM pattern carried by a wave packet does not represent the stimulus to other parts of the brain. It carries the relevant knowledge about the stimulus for integration with wave packets from other sensory cortices, both directly to other sensory and motor cortices and through the limbic system, ultimately to form a unified macroscopic concept as the culmination of an act of perception with closure of the action-perception cycle by extrapolation to prediction of a new future state.

The reflex model originated in the Cartesian metaphor likening the flow of spirit in brain operations to hydrodynamics. Descartes conceived the *sensorium communum* as a complex mirror under central control. The metaphor persists today when brain operations are likened to information processing in computers.

The action-perception model originated over 400 years before Descartes in Thomas Aquinas' description of intention ("intendere" from the Latin word for bow string, hence tendon) (Aquinas, 1272) by which brain operations thrust the body into its surround and acquired knowledge by adaptation ("adequatio") to the environment. Goal-oriented behaviors have been described repeatedly in the 20th century by pragmatists (Dewey, 1914), developmental psychologists (Piaget, 1930; Köhler, 1940), existentialists

(Merleau-Ponty, 1945) and enactionists (Clark, 1996), however without benefit of nonlinear brain dynamics. Only in recent years have developments in dynamics and field theory provided the concepts required to model large-scale neural activity: scale-free dynamics (Breakspear, 2004; Chen and Shi, 2004; Freeman, 2006a, 2006b), circular causality (Haken, 1983), stabilization of brains in pseudo-equilibrium at self-organized criticality (Jensen, 1998), dissipative structures forming by phase transitions far from thermodynamic equilibrium (Prigogine, 1980), anomalous dispersion in the dissemination of phase transitions (Freeman, 2000), extensions of random graph theory into 'neuropercolation' (Kozma et al., 2005), and repetitive destabilization of cortical dynamics in spontaneous symmetry breaking as described in many-body physics (Freeman and Vitiello, 2006, 2007).

4. The Construction and Expression of Knowledge through Background Activity

Even the most casual observations of the electric and magnetic fields of the action potentials and dendritic waves from normal brains reveal the spontaneous background activity. Stimulus-response determinists treat this activity as noise and remove it by averaging in order to retrieve event-related potentials (ERP) as signals. Neurodynamicists by close examination of the background activity have extracted and displayed significant mesoscopic structures in the background activity (Figure 2).

The individual pulses in trains of action potentials from cortical neurons are uncorrelated within themselves and among others and can be described as a random walk (Kozma et al., 2005) except for the refractory periods. When summed over neighborhoods with ~10^4 neurons their combined activity conforms to Brown noise (Schroeder, 1991) with Gaussian amplitude density distributions and spectra of log power vs. log frequency with slopes near -2 ("$1/f^2$") but falling to -3 or steeper in slow-wave sleep (Freeman, 2006a). The activity has been demonstrated to be generated by mutual excitation (positive feedback) among cortical excitatory neurons that is stabilized by the absolute and relative refractory periods (Freeman, 1975) and is therefore governed by a point attractor (Freeman, 2007). These features carry over into the dendritic potentials through a low pass filter contributed by the passive membrane time constants of dendritic membranes and their cable properties. Negative feedback from inhibitory neurons operates like a band pass filter to introduce oscillations giving the EEG peaks in the spectrum in the beta (12-30 Hz) and gamma (30-80 Hz) ranges.

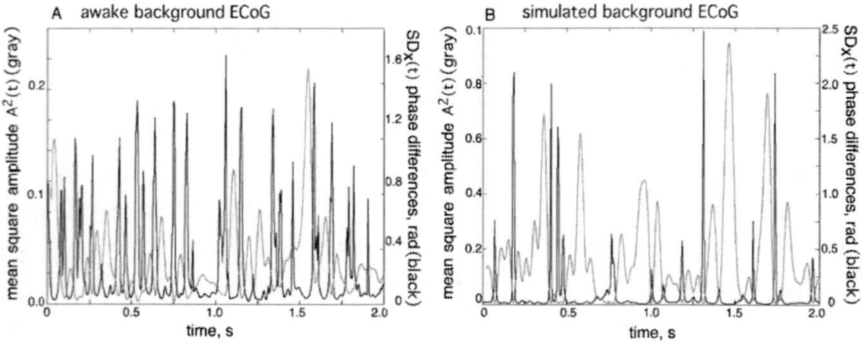

Figure 2. A. This is an example of the analytic signal from array recording of ECoG from a human subject at rest, showing the background activity. When the spatial standard deviation of phase differences, $SD_X(t)$, falls to a low value, the mean analytic amplitude, $\underline{A}(t)$, increases to a maximum during the period of relatively constant frequency that follows a phase transition (Freeman, 2004b). B. This pattern is simulated by passing *brown noise* ($1/f^2$) through a band pass filter in the gamma range, which shows that the background activity conforms to Rayleigh noise (Freeman, 1975). Mean analytic amplitude and spatial variance of analytic phase co-vary inversely (Freeman, 2006). The properties of the background noise and the occurrence of the null spikes at which the analytic phase is undefined can only be explained by field theory. From Freeman (2007).

The oscillations recur in bursts separated by intermittent epochs of severe abatement of background noise amplitude ("null spikes", Figure 2) that recur at rates in the theta (3-7 Hz) and alpha (7-12 Hz) ranges (Freeman, 2006a). These null spikes in the background activity are best seen in the analytic signals derived with the Hilbert transform (Freeman, 2006c) applied to electrocorticograms (ECoG) recorded with arrays of electrodes implanted directly onto the cortical surface of brains in animals (Freeman, 2004a,b) and humans (Freeman et al., 2006). They have also been demonstrated in the scalp EEG in normal subjects (Freeman, et al., 2003; Freeman, Burke and Holmes, 2003). These null spikes are frequency-specific for the beta and gamma ranges that are determined by the delays in the feedback pathways, local feedback with shorter delays giving gamma (Freeman, 1975) and global feedback with longer delays giving beta.

The amplitudes of the background activity increase with increased arousal and motivation (hunger, fear, etc.). During the bursts between null spikes there emerge spatial patterns of amplitude modulation (AM) of beta-gamma oscillatory wave packets that recur at frequencies in the theta-alpha ranges (Freeman, Burke and Holmes, 2003; Freeman, 2005a). The AM patterns in the brains of animals are correlated with the actions and inferred perceptions of the animals, but as noted earlier the patterns lack invariance with respect to conditioned stimuli. For example, animals conditioned to discriminate between a reinforced and an unreinforced conditioned stimulus develop three classes of AM patterns, one for each stimulus and one for the background. When the reinforcement is switched, all three AM patterns change slightly but significantly (Freeman and Grajski, 1987). Therefore, the fields are not fixed representations of the stimuli; they express knowledge about the situations that the animals have learned to expect by interactions with their environments, knowledge that continually evolves with each new sample in changing contexts. The AM patterns of wave packets are created by self-organizing brain dynamics based on synapses among cortical neurons that are modified by prior and on-going learning. The AM fields in each sensory cortex form sequences of stationary states that resemble frames in a cinema (Sacks, 2004). Each frame is separated from those preceding and following by a phase transition that imposes a discontinuity in cortical dynamics, a discontinuity that appears to be facilitated by the null spike in the background activity. These data show that the cognitively related content of AM patterns is not superimposed on the background, from which it can be retrieved by averaging over trials. The content is created when sensory input during a null spike activates a nerve cell assembly that accesses an attractor, which re-structures the background activity as it returns by imposing its AM pattern (Freeman, 2007). The transition constitutes the retrieval of knowledge guided by the stimulus, not the processing of information contained in the stimulus.

Two classes of AM pattern have been found in animals trained in classical and operant conditioning paradigms. In each trial early after stimulus onset an AM pattern appears that is modality-specific; its mesoscopic field is localized in the relevant primary sensory area, and the oscillation has a carrier frequency in the gamma range. Later but before the response onset another type of oscillatory macroscopic field appears that is synchronized over all of the primary sensory areas and the entorhinal cortex (Freeman and Rogers, 2003). The frequency is in the beta range, and all sensory and limbic areas participate in its AM pattern (Freeman and Burke, 2003). Gamma oscillations seldom occur in prestimulus control epochs, whereas beta oscillations occur with the same probability in prestimulus and poststimulus epochs.

The proposed sequence of events in an action-perception cycle is summarized as follows. The expression of intent to act by initiating a sniff, whisk or saccade is accompanied by an update by corollary discharges of the attractor landscapes in all sensory and motor areas. Each area has its own asynchronous pacing of opportunities for phase transitions in the null spikes in its background activity. The arrival of a corollary discharge may precipitate a macroscopic phase transition that is manifested in a beta burst. The arrival of a volley of action potentials relayed from sensory receptors, when it coincides with a local null spike in the gamma range, achieves the signal-to-noise ratio that is required for the selection of a nerve cell assembly, thereby accessing the corresponding attractor by a mesoscopic phase transition. When the background noise returns, the gamma band contains a wave packet with the AM pattern corresponding to the class to which the stimulus is assigned in each modality. The sensory cortices broadcast their wave packets to widespread targets; the signals converge by stages to the outer layers of the entorhinal cortex, go through the hippocampal loop, and return to the inner layers of the entorhinal cortex, whereupon the combined signals are sent back to all of the sensory areas. As described above the subsequent beta AM patterns are synchronized across sensory and limbic cortices (Freeman and Rogers, 2003) and are polysensory, because classification is optimal when EEG information from visual, auditory, somatic, olfactory, and entorhinal areas is included, and it is diminished when any of these components is omitted (Freeman and Burke, 2003).

These data indicate that, roughly half a second after stimulus onset, two to three stimulus-related macroscopic cortical AM patterns of synchronized oscillation emerge preceding the onset of a response to a stimulus, each lasting on the order of a tenth of a second. In cats and rabbits the correlation distance suffices to extend across the entire hemisphere (Freeman, 2004a); in human scalp EEG the correlation distance occasionally reaches the length of the recording array (189 mm) for EEG (Freeman, Burke and Holmes, 2003) and an estimated 225 mm for MEG (Bassett et al., 2006). It is a subset of these macroscopic patterns that I propose as a neural correlate of consciousness. What is not yet known is whether the large domains form either a mosaic of discrete patches interacting as a network, in accord with a Newtonian model, or a continuum as in a Faraday-Maxwell field. Wolfgang Köhler (1940) was quite explicit about this: "Our present knowledge of human perception leaves no doubt as to the general form of any theory which is to do justice to such knowledge: a theory of perception must be a field theory. By this we mean that the neural functions and processes with which the perceptual facts are associated in each case are located in a continuous medium" p 55). Regrettably Köhler identified his perceptual field with the epiphenomenal electric field of the EEG, of which the Coulomb forces are much too weak to synchronize the observed oscillations in wave packets (Freeman and Baird, 1989). This subsidiary hypothesis was easily disproved by Sperry (1958) and Pribram (1971), with the unfortunate outcome that field hypotheses were largely abandoned by mainstream neuroscientists.

5. Deducing Some Properties of Consciousness from Nonlinear Brain Dynamics

Since I cannot demonstrate what my subjects experience or even whether they are conscious, I describe consciousness as existing in the state of engagement with the environment that may be experienced by animals and pre-lingual children who cannot speak about it. This state that one can attribute to engaged subjects can be behaviorally distinguished from states on the one hand of self-awareness, introspection, or 'spectatoring' and on the other hand of dozing, dreaming, deep anesthesia, and *absence* in partial complex seizure. I define three neural correlates of the designated state in animals: arousal, intention, and attention. The degree of arousal (conceived by psychologists in terms of motivation, drive or desire) can be estimated by the mean level of self-stabilized background spike firing and dendritic activity (Freeman, 2007), for example, by measuring the root mean square amplitude of gamma activity from the olfactory cortex (Freeman, 1960, 1975). The degree of intention (often conflated by psychologists with motivation) can be estimated by the *a priori* likelihood that any one of a list of designated responses will occur following delivery of a learned stimulus, and by an index, $H_e(t)$, defined as pragmatic information (Freeman, 2004a,b) that is calculated from the analytic signal of neocortical EEG (Freeman, 2005a). The degree of attention is more problematic, owing to the lack of a commonly accepted neural referent. According to James (1890): "Everyone knows what attention is. Focalization, concentration, of consciousness is of its essence. It implies withdrawal from some things in order to deal effectively with others, and is a condition which has a real opposite in the confused, dazed, scatterbrained state." A more contemporary dictionary definition of attention is "An adjustment of the sense organs and of the organism generally, preparatory to actual observation of something; a focusing of conscious activity on anything; as, attention to a problem; the act or fact of bringing something into clear awareness; …" (Webster, 2nd ed., unabridged, 1949). In Newtonian models the degree of attention can be assessed by the synchronization of firing of tuned neurons (Mehta, Ulbert and Schroeder, 2000; Posner and Dehaene, 1994). In field models the neurally based measure of the level of attention may be indexed by the degree complexity of attractor landscapes in the sensory cortices that serve to predict expected classes of sensory input, as measured by multivariate classification algorithms applied to AM patterns (Viana Di Prisco, 1985; Barrie, Freeman and Lenhart, 1996; Kay and Freeman, 1998; Ohl, Scheich and Freeman, 2001; Kozma and Freeman, 2002; Freeman, 2005a). The landscapes are based in nerve cell assemblies formed in cortical neuropil during cumulative learning. The precise numbers and locations of modified synapses cannot be directly observed or measured. Their existence is demonstrated by the short-latency emergence of gamma AM patterns following receipt by subjects of relevant conditioned stimuli.

At what stage of the action-perception cycle might consciousness emerge? While involvement of the hippocampal formation is not wholly necessary for consciousness in the limited sense here intended, it is necessary for the accumulation of episodic memories into the recollection of a lifetime (Squires, 1990), and since such memories typically are polymodal, and since human subjects require roughly half a second before reporting awareness of a stimulus (Libet, 1994), a candidate for the neural correlate of consciousness on perceiving a stimulus is one or more of the beta macroscopic events recorded late in the stimulus-response interval. Adequate EEG data from human experiments in self-awareness are not yet on hand. Which in a sequence of beta frames the correlate might be identified with is not clear; that cannot be determined from tests with non-human animals, because they lack speech. The further problem is that turbulent streams of multiple overlapping spatial patterns of phase and amplitude in beta oscillations flow equally before and after the arrival of an expected stimulus. The durations of the patterns give power-law distributions with means and variances that change with the duration of the measuring window (Freeman, 2004b; Freeman et al., 2006). The patterns resemble bubbles in a pan of boiling water that maintain its critical temperature, and the avalanches in a sand pile that maintain its critical angle. In cortex this on-going activity manifests the maintenance by cortex of its conditionally stable level of activity at self-organized criticality, for which the self-maintained critical variable is the self-regulated mean level of cortical firing (Freeman, 2007). The deviations from the power-law distributions of spectral energy in subjects at rest, which manifests endogenous noise, is the emergence in the cortices of engaged subjects of local peaks of spectral energy reflecting oscillatory bursts carrying spatial AM patterns that last longer than expected for noise and therefore reveal signals (Freeman. 2005). And among these self-organized bubbles are synchronized oscillations in the beta and possibly gamma ranges that rapidly form and dissolve with correlation distances at least 189 mm (Freeman, Burke and Holmes, 2003) and 225 mm (Bassett et al., 2006), which may be requisite for the apparent unity of consciousness.

This excess of long-lasting AM patterns having 3-5 cycles of the carrier frequency includes the AM patterns that are classifiable with respect to conditioned stimuli. They comprise a small proportion of the concomitant AM patterns, which might include not only percepts of stimuli but also motor commands, corollary discharges, and expectations that are likely to be unconscious or preconscious. In the view from neurodynamics the identity of an individual, the “real person”, “proto-self” (Damasio, 1999) or “global work space” (Baars, 1997) is embodied in the entirety of the brain-body dynamics, not only in the fragments available to introspection. The prime source of self-knowledge and being known by others is observation and inspection of one’s actions, not one’s stated intentions. Voluntary actions might be classed as those relatively few intentional actions that succeed informed reflection without necessarily conforming to its conclusion (Davidson, 1980); intentional actions lacking this condition are thereby not conscious. EEG evidence (Walter, 1953; Libet, 1994) indicates that voluntary actions are initiated about half a second before awareness of the intent to act, leaving time for veto.

The veto is obviously by intention, which is the mechanism described above for the action-perception cycle. It is unclear what the timing might be for the preconscious perception of an event *vs.* the decision to report the perception *vs.* the awareness of deciding. While in principle the AM patterns of beta wave packets may be accessed through the scalp EEG, the techniques for doing so remain to be developed in human studies. Several experimental findings give reason to expect eventual success. First, intentional actions involve the whole body (Bernstein, 1967), even for constrained actions such as finger-presses, owing in the latter case to active inhibition of all other movements, to anticipatory feedforward set-ups for exteroceptive and proprioceptive feedback, and to the janitorial back-ups in posture, autonomic adaptations and neuroendocrine regulation, so that cortical fields of the relevant macroscopic beta events are likely spread widely and involve the frontal and parietal lobes. Second, the dynamics of neocortex is scale-free (Freeman, 2006b), meaning that the time required for reorganization in a phase transition is independent of the size of the domain of incipient synchrony, so they may be immense compared to the radii of dendritic branches. Third, the spatial resolution of amplitude differences carried by beta-gamma activity fields may approach the dimensions of gyri (1-3 cm) (Freeman et al., 2003), indicating that the most revealing spacing of electrodes (the Nyquist sampling rate) on the scalp might be 3-5 mm, not the 25-50 mm currently in common clinical use. Fourth, the information that contributes to classification is equal on all electrodes in an array; the finding is that no channel is more or less important than any other; the implication is that classification improves with the number of electrodes irrespective of location, provided the locations are not moved between samples.

Some further properties that can be deduced from dynamics and field potential data are that consciousness is reactive and judgmental of the results of intentional action late in the action-perception cycle, not enactive in the initiation of an act: "What have I done?" rather than "What shall I do?" In this perspective its role is to defer action pending closure of the search of knowledge from experience prior to an intentional action. Judgment consists in constructing and contrasting possible courses of action given the environmental circumstances of the moment. When a conclusion is reached on what is best done, action ensues, but all too often the action initiated is not that considered as optimal but may be detrimental. Davidson (1980) described this type of action as 'incontinent'; it is clear evidence that the conscious state, whatever it might be, is not the same as the neural activity pattern that actually selects the action initiated.

Conclusion

While neurodynamics cannot explain consciousness, it does open novel perspectives for discussion, and it offers four predictions of neural correlates of consciousness that follow from a field theory and that cannot be explained by current network theories. To be a field in the sense intended, a cooperative domain must be an embedding continuum that provides energy at every point, as distinct from a network of synchronized nodes such as synapses and trigger zones at which energy is conceived as a point process. The embedding field is apparent in the background activity, which is highly structured by diffuse interactions (Figure 2). The carrier oscillations must have a spatial structure of analytic phase modulation indicating that cortex is a relativistic medium as distinct from 'zero lag' synchrony (Figure 1). And the neural correlate of a reported experience must be an AM pattern in which highs and lows have equal information, as distinct from a code in which the amount of information is related to the intensity of activity of each neuron in a focus: its frequency or timing of firing viewed a point process.

From these considerations I propose that consciousness can be defined as a field of force that is centered in a brain and that operates through the body simultaneously into all levels of the surround from subatomic to social. Awareness is perception of the forces of self and others as in peer pressures and familial forces. Unconsciousness comprises the immense reservoir that is provided by the nonlinear neurodynamics of the neural interactions, and that shapes the contents and structures of the field of force.

We perceive that kind of force in the same way that we perceive all kinds of force — gravitational, electric, magnetic, chemical, thermal, social — through volitional actions of the body and their impacts on our sensory and perceptual systems.

We describe and measure that kind of force in the same way that we measure all kinds of force: indirectly by measurement of the correlates of that force in the patterns of goal-directed bodily motion and acceleration of mass in space and time, i.e., intentional behavior.

This definition is consistent *inter alia* with the views of Aquinas, James, Dewey, Freud, Köhler, Koffka, Lotka, Merleau-Ponty, and with the Chinese conception of Qi. Owing to lack of sufficient data, this definition is at present limited to consciousness in animals, infants, and pre-lingual children. Unlike Whitehead (1938), Penrose (1994) and Chalmers (1996) I do not postulate panpsychism but restrict consciousness to animals having advanced laminated neuropil (cortex), which has evolved three times independently in earth's history, resulting in the diverse brain structures in highly intelligent species in three phyla: Mollusca (cuttlefish), Arthropoda (honeybees), and Vertebrata (humans).

Brain science takes us beyond our philosophical predecessors into mind science. From measurements of neural correlates of behavior, I deduce the following properties of consciousness from its conception as a field of force:

- Brains hold themselves at criticality, where all frequencies and wavelengths coexist in scale-free fields of neural activity, directing the brain-body system to move unitarily and instantly in any selected direction. This is an up-date and extension of the classic Sherringtonian concept of "the final common path".

- Discontinuities: The stream of consciousness is not continuous; it is in cinematographic frames formed by endogenous phase transitions that are enabled by the property of criticality.
- Arousal: The neural correlate is the mean firing rate of neurons throughout the cortex, sampled through its control parameter, the strength of dendritic current manifested in the brain waves. Modeling with differential equations or equivalent is required.
- Attention: The neural correlate is the set of attractor landscapes in the phase space of the primary sensory cortices. Again, modeling with nonlinear equations is required.
- Intention: The neural correlate is the identification of spatiotemporal patterns of beta and gamma activity in cinematographic frames correlated with goal-directed behaviors. The tools of multivariate statistics, engineering mathematics, and physics are required.
- The role of consciousness is deferral of future action pending closure of evaluation of the information acquired by prior intentional action: stop and think.

The aim of consciousness studies should be a set of master equations that relate material and psychosocial state variables, comparable to the equations of Newton, Maxwell and Einstein, but going beyond the physical aspects of the universe and unifying it with the human aspects of the universe. Such a mind theory is needed to provide a scientific foundation for the behavioral sciences, including psychiatry, as envisioned by Freud (1895).

References

Arianrhod R (2005) *Einstein's Heroes. Imagining the World through the Language of Mathematics*. Oxford UK; Oxford U.P.

Baars BJ (1997) *In the Theater of Consciousness: The Workspace of the Mind*. New York: Oxford UP.

Barlow HB (1972) Single units and sensation: A neuron doctrine for perceptual psychology? *Perception* **1:** 371-394.

Barrett TW (2000) Topology and the physical properties of the electromagnetic field. *Apeiron* **7**: 3-11.

Barrett TW (2001) Topological approaches to electromagnetism. In: Evans M (ed.) *Modern Nonlinear Optics*, 2nd ed. New York:, Wiley Interscience, pp. 699-734.

Barrie JM, Freeman WJ and Lenhart M (1996) Modulation by discriminative training of spatial patterns of gamma EEG amplitude and phase in neocortex of rabbits. *J. Neurophysiol.* **76**: 520-539.

Bartlett Sir FC (1932) *Remembering.* Cambridge UK: Cambridge University Press.

Bassett DS, Meyer-Lindenberg A, Achard S, Duke T and Bullmore E (2006) Adaptive reconfiguration of fractal small-world human brain functional networks. *PNAS*, **103**: 19518–19523.

Bernstein N (1967) *The Coordination and Regulation of Movements.* (trans. Drillis RJ). New York: Pergamon Press.

Breakspear M (2004) Dynamic connectivity in neural systems: Theoretical and empirical considerations. *Neuroinformatics* **2**(2): 205-225.

Chalmers DJ (1996) The Conscious Mind. *In Search of a Fundamental Theory.* New York: Oxford University Press.

Chapline G (1999) Is theoretical physics the same thing as mathematics? *Physical Reports* **315**: 95-10.

Chen Q and Shi D (2004) The modeling of scale-free networks. *Physica A* **333**: 240-248.

Clark A (1996) *Being There. Putting Brain, Body, and World Together Again.* Cambridge MA: MIT Press.

Damaso AR (1999) *The Feeling of What Happens: Body, Emotion and the Making of Consciousness.* London UK: Vintage.

Davidson D (1980) Actions, reasons, and causes. In: *Essays on Actions and Events*. Oxford UK: Clarendon Press.

Dewey J (1914) Psychological doctrine in philosophical teaching. *J. Philos.* **11**: 505-512.

Engel AK, Kreiter AK, König P and Singer W (1991) Synchronization of oscillatory neuronal responses between striate and extrastriate visual cortical areas of the cat. *Proc. Nat. Acad. Sci. USA* **88**: 6048-6052.

Ferster CB and Skinner BF (1957) *Schedules of Reinforcement*. Englewood Cliffs NJ: Prentice-Hall.

Freeman WJ (1960) Correlation of electrical activity of prepyriform cortex and behavior in cat. *J. Neurophysiol.* **23**: 111-131.

Freeman WJ (1975) *Mass Action in the Nervous System*. New York: Academic. Electronic 2004: http://sulcus.berkeley.edu/MANSWWW/MANSWWW.html

Freeman WJ (2000) *Neurodynamics: An Exploration of Mesoscopic Brain Dynamics*, London UK: Springer.

Freeman WJ (2004a) Origin, structure, and role of background EEG activity. Part 1. Analytic amplitude. *Clin. Neurophysiol.* **115**: 2077-2088.

Freeman WJ (2004b) Origin, structure, and role of background EEG activity. Part 2. Analytic phase. *Clin. Neurophysiol.* **115**: 2089-2107.

Freeman WJ (2005a) Origin, structure, and role of background EEG activity. Part 3. Neural frame classification. *Clin. Neurophysiol.* **116** 5): 1118-1129.

Freeman WJ (2005b) NDN, volume transmission, and self-organization in brain dynamics. *J. Integrative Neuroscience* **4** (4): 407-421.

Freeman WJ (2006a) Origin, structure, and role of background EEG activity. Part 4. Neural frame simulation. *Clin. Neurophysiol.* **117**: 572-589.

Freeman WJ (2006b) Scale-free neocortical dynamics. *Encyc Comp Neurosci,* Izhikevich E (ed.). http://www.scholarpedia.org/article/Scale-free_neocortical_dynamics

Freeman WJ (2006c) Hilbert transform for brain waves. *Encyc Comp Neurosci,* Izhikevich E (ed.) http://www.scholarpedia.org/article/Hilbert_transform_for brain_waves

Freeman WJ (2007) Proposed cortical 'shutter' in cinematographic perception. Ch. In: *Neurodynamics of Cognition and Consciousness*. Kozma R and Perlovsky L (eds.). New York: Springer, pp. 11-38.

Freeman WJ and Baird B (1987) Relation of olfactory EEG to behavior: Spatial analysis: *Behav. Neurosci.* **101**:393-408.

Freeman WJ and Baird B (1989) Effects of applied electric current fields on cortical neural activity. Chapter in: Schwartz E (ed.) *Computational Neuroscience*. New York, Plenum Press. pp. 274-287.

Freeman WJ and Burke BC (2003) A neurobiological theory of meaning in perception. Part 4. Multicortical patterns of amplitude modulation in gamma EEG. *Int. J. Bifurc. Chaos* **13**: 2857-2866.

Freeman WJ, Burke BC, Holmes MD and Vanhatalo S (2003) Spatial spectra of scalp EEG and EMG from awake humans. *Clin. Neurophysiol*. **114**: 1055-1060. http://repositories.
cdlib.org/postprints/989

Freeman WJ, Burke BC and Holmes MD (2003) Aperiodic phase re-setting in scalp EEG of beta-gamma oscillations by state transitions at alpha-theta rates. *Human Brain Mapping* **19**(4): 248-272.

Freeman WJ and Grajski KA (1987) Relation of olfactory EEG to behavior: Factor analysis: *Behav. Neurosci.* **101**: 766-777.

Freeman WJ, Holmes MD, West GA and Vanhatalo S (2006) Fine spatiotemporal structure of phase in human intracranial EEG. *Clin. Neurophysiol*. **117** (6): 1228-1243.

Freeman WJ and Rogers LJ (2003) A neurobiological theory of meaning in perception. Part 5. Multicortical patterns of phase modulation in gamma EEG. *Int. J. Bifurc Chaos* **13**: 2867-2887.

Freeman WJ and Vitiello G (2006) Nonlinear brain dynamics as macroscopic manifestation of underlying many-body field dynamics. *Physics of Life Reviews* **3**: 93-118.

Freeman WJ and Vitiello G (2007) The dissipative quantum model of brain and laboratory observations. *Electronic J. Theoretical. Physics* **4**, 1-18.

Freud S (1895) The project of a scientific psychology. Chapter in: *The Origins of Psycho-Analysis.* Bonaparte M, Freud A, Kris E (eds.), Mosbacher E, Strachey J (trans.). New York: Basic Books, 1954.

Gibson JJ (1979) *The Ecological Approach to Visual Perception*. Boston: Houghton Mifflin.

Haken H (1983) *Synergetics: An Introduction*. Berlin: Springer-Verlag.

Harnad S (1999) The symbol grounding problem. *Physica D* **42**: 445-346.

Houk JC (2005) Agents of the mind. *Biol. Cybern.* **92**: 427-437.

James W (1890) *The Principles of Psychology*. New York: Henry Holt.

Jensen HJ (1998) *Self-Organized Criticality: Emergent Complex Behavior in Physical and Biological Systems*. New York: Cambridge UP.

Jibu M, Pribram KH and Yasue K (1996) From conscious experience to memory storage and retrieval: the role of quantum brain dynamics and boson condensation of evanescent photons. *Intern. J. Modern. Physics B* **10** (13 and 14): 1735-1754.
John ER (2001) A field theory of consciousness. *Consciousness and Cognition* 10: 184-213.
Kay LM and Freeman WJ (1998) Bidirectional processing in the olfactory-limbic axis during olfactory behavior. *Behav. Neurosci.* **112**: 541-553.
Köhler W (1940) *Dynamics in Psychology*. New York NY: Grove Press.
Kozma R and Freeman WJ (2001) Chaotic resonance: Methods and applications for robust classification of noisy and variable patterns. *Intern. J. Bifurc. Chaos* **10**: 2307-2322.
Kozma R and Freeman WJ (2002) Classification of EEG patterns using nonlinear dynamics and identifying chaotic phase transitions. *Neurocomputing* **44**: 1107-1112.
Kozma R and Freeman WJ (2003) Basic principles of the KIV model and its application to the navigation problem. *J. Integrative Neurosci* **2**: 125-145.
Kozma R, Freeman WJ and Erdí P (2003) The KIV model – nonlinear spatio-temporal dynamics of the primordial vertebrate forebrain. *Neurocomputing* **52**: 819-826.
Kozma R, Puljic M, Balister P, Bollobas B and Freeman WJ (2004) Neuropercolation: A Random Cellular Automata Approach to Spatio-Temporal Neurodynamics. Ch. in: *Lecture Notes in Computer Science*: **141**.225.40.170 springerlink.com
Kuhn TS (1962) *The Structure of Scientific Revolutions*. Chicago: Univ. Chicago Press.
Libet B (1994) *Neurophysiology of Consciousness: Selected Papers and New Essays*. Boston MA: Birkhauser.
Lucky RW (1989) *Silicon Dreams: Information, Man and Machine*. New York: St. Martin's Press.
Mehta AD, Ulbert I and Schroeder CE (2000) Intermodal selective attention in monkeys. I: Distribution and timing of effects across visual areas. *Cerebral Cortex* **10**(4): 343-358.
Melloni L, Molina C, Pena M, Torres D, Singer W and Rodriguez E (2007) Synchronization of neural activity across cortical areas correlates with conscious perception. *J. Neurosci.* **270**(11): 2858-2865.
Merleau-Ponty M (1942/1963) *The Structure of Behavior* (Fischer AL, Trans.). Boston: Beacon Press.
Merleau-Ponty M (1945/1962) *Phenomenology of Perception,* (C Smith, trans.). New York: Humanities Press.
Ohl FW, Scheich H and Freeman WJ (2001) Change in pattern of ongoing cortical activity with auditory category learning. *Nature* **412**: 733-736.
Penrose R (1994) *Shadows of the Mind*. Oxford UK: Oxford University Press.
Posner MI, Dehaene S (1994) Attentional networks. *Trends Neurosci* **17**(2): 75-79.
Piaget J (1930) The Child's Conception of Physical Causality. New York: Harcourt, Brace.
Pribram KH (1971) *Languages of the Brain*: *Experimental Paradoxes and Principles in Neuropsychology*. Englewood Cliffs, NJ: Prentice-Hall.
Pribram KH (1991) *Brain and Perception: Holonomy and Structure in Figural Processing*. New Jersey: Lawrence Erlbaum Assoc.
Prigogine I (1980) *From Being to Becoming: Time and Complexity in the Physical Sciences*. WH Freeman: San Francisco.

Principe JC, Tavares VG, Harris JG and Freeman WJ (2001) Design and implementation of a biologically realistic olfactory cortex in analog VLSI. *Proc IEEE* **89**: 1030-1051.

Sacks O (2004) In the river of consciousness. *New York Review* **51**: Number 1, January 15.

Schillen TB and König P (1994) Binding by temporal structure in multiple feature domains on an oscillatory neuronal network. *Biol. Cybern* **70**: 397-405.

Schroeder M (1991) *Fractals, Chaos*, Power Laws. San Francisco: WH Freeman.

Searle JR (1995) The Mystery of Consciousness. *New York Review* 2-18 November

Skarda CA and Freeman WJ (1987) How brains make chaos in order to make sense of the world, *Behavioral and Brain Sci.* **10**: 161-195.

Sperry RW (1950) Neural basis of the spontaneous optokinetic response. *J. Comp. Physiol.* **43**: 482-489.

Sperry RW (1958) Physiological plasticity and brain circuit theory. In: Harlow HF, Woolsey CN (eds.) *Biological and Biochemical Bases of Behavior*. Madison WI: Univ Wisconsin Press.

Squires E (1990) *Conscious Mind in the Physical* World. Bristol UK: Adam Hilger.

Taylor JG (2003) Paying Attention to Consciousness. *Prog. Neurobiol.* **71**:305-335.

Tononi G, Edelman GM. (2000) *A Universe of Consciousness*. New York: Basic Books.

Viana Di Prisco G, Freeman WJ (1985) Odor-related bulbar EEG spatial pattern analysis during appetitive conditioning in rabbits. *Behavioral Neuroscience* **99**: 962-978.

von Holst E and Mittelstädt H (1950) Das Reafferenzprinzip. Wechselwirkung zwischen Zentralnervensystem und Peripherie. *Naturwissenschaften* **37**: 464-476.

Walter WG (1953) *The Living Brain*. New York: W. W. Norton.

Weiskrantz L (1998) Consciousness and commentaries. In: Hameroff SR, Kaszriak A, Scott AC (eds.), *Toward a Science of Consciousness II*. Cambridge MA: MIT Press, pp. 371-377.

Whitehead AN (1938) *Modes of Thought*. New York: Macmillan.

Chapter 3

Circle Mapping Applied in Neural Impulse Sequence Analysis—Neuron Code Research*

Qinye Tong[1,2,3,†], Lunping Fang[1], Hong Zhang[1,2,3], Mingqi Qian[2,3], Xu Li[3] and Xiaobeng Han[3]

[1]Center of Neural Information Research, Zhejiang University, Hangzhou, Zhejiang, China
[2]Key Laboratory of Biomedical Engineering Ministry of Education, Zhejiang University, Hangzhou, Zhejiang, China
[3]Department of Biomedical Engineering, Zhejiang University, Hangzhou, Zhejiang, China

Abstract

In neural network, neurons usually work above the threshold taking the form of impulse sequence, which is termed action potential in electrophysiology, except for a few neurons in sensory organ working below the threshold.

In the neural network, a train of impulses will change to another train of impulses via one unit always, therefore the whole neural network can be called "pulsed neural network".

Here, the basic unit involved is: A neuron, which is fed simultaneously by the outputs of some neurons through the synapses, will generate another impulse sequence (output). Then the question comes: what regularity underlies between the input and output? Can impulse sequence serve as coding of neural information?

---

* This article was originally published in Chaos and Complexity Letters, volume 4 number 2 (2010).

† Corresponding Author's Email: bitong@public.zju.edu.cn.

In: Neuroscience and Technology Transform the Educational Ecosystem
Editors: Franco F. Orsucci and Nicoletta Sala
ISBN: 979-8-88697-157-6

In our opinion, before we can confirm that the neural impulse sequence is neural information coding, we have to answer the following questions: (1) Is the neural impulse sequence space an ordered space? (2) Are there any features of operation or mapping in the neural impulse sequence space?

In this article, Circle mapping together with symbolic dynamics method is used to solve the problems mentioned above. It forms a base for the research of neural impulse information coding.

1. Introduction[1]

Gilles Laurent wrote an article in SCIENCE [1], beginning with "Studying a neural code requires asking specific questions, such as the following: What information do the signals carry? What formats are used? Why are such formats used? Although superficially unambiguous, such questions are charged with hidden difficulties and biases". Eric R. Kandel also published article [2] in SCIENCE, expressing that modern neural science is in the irrational state.

Frankly speaking, neural impulse sequence should be neural information coding. However, no people can describe it clearly, and they don't know the meaning of the train of impulses. Some people even think that a single train of impulses implies nothing.

Therefore many hypothesis, such as mean firing rates（rat code） [3, 4], distributing function [5, 6] (temporal code), neural ensemble theory (population code) [1, 7, 8] and etc, are proposed. In our opinion, before we can confirm that the neural impulse sequence is neural information coding, we have to solve the following problems:

1.1. Is the Impulse Sequence Space an Ordered One?

If all impulse sequences there are all in the neural system combined to form an impulse sequence space Ω, then Ω must be an ordered space. Because magnitude is one important characteristic of all input signal of neural system, for instance, the light accepted by people's eyes may be bright or dim, sound

[1] Supported by the Dedicated Pre-studied of the National Basic Research Program (973 Program) (under grant No.2002CCA01800) & Natural Science Foundation Program (under grant No. 30170267).

accepted by people's ear may be loud or low, and scents accepted by people's nose may be strong or weak, To represent external signal by neural impulse it is required that Ω should be an ordered space when to build a corresponding relationship between neural impulse sequence and external stimulus, or at least, a subspace in Ω space is ordered.

1.2. Are There the Characteristics of Operation and Mapping in Ω Space?

It is well known that man's neural system does have ability of information processing. And information processing relies on transformation and mapping. If Ω space becomes a coding space, it must possess the property of operation.

Suppose that η_i is an element of Ω, namely, a train of impulse,

$$\Omega = \{\eta_i\} \tag{1}$$

It's the question to explore which the characteristics Ω has. Just as set theory exposes, some sets can become a group (such as Renormalization group, Galois group and so on); some set can make up a ring (such as ring of integers and so on) or algebra (such as Boolean algebra, Lie algebra and so on).

Then what system can Ω make up of? What transformation can be performed in Ω?

Though EEG signal contains information, people have not discovered that transformation can be performed in EEG set or ordering operation can be implemented, which makes it impossible for EEG signal to be utilized as coding of neural information.

If the above two problems are not solved, the research on neural informatics will be seriously hindered.

For neural network, only a few neurons in sensory organ work below the threshold, the generated potential of which is called localized graded potential in electrophysiology.

And other neurons all work above the threshold with the form of impulse sequence (hight action potential).

In neural network, a train of impulse will change to another train of impulse via one unit, therefore the whole neural network can be called "spiking neural network".

Here, the basic procedure can be described that the neuron, which is linked simultaneously with several other neurons by their synapses, will be stimulated by their outputs to generate another impulse sequence. Here comes the question: what is the relationship between the input and output? This article uses circle mapping to analyze this problem, and solution to the two questions above is gradually approached.

2. Circle Mapping Based Analysis on Output Impulse from Neuron

Circle mapping of neuron is a necessary theoretical tool in proving whether Ω is an ordered space, understanding the regularity of information (i.e., trains of neural spikes) change, and disclosing the principle of neural coding [9, 10].

First, let us consider the response when one neuron is under the stimulation of a constant frequency. The classical H-H model (2) is used to describe the potential change of neuron. Many people have contributed improvements to H-H model in recent years, however, we think that these modifications to the model are in quantity, and have not been involved in quality. From the late analysis, it can be seen that it will not lose generality if H-H model is used for discussion.

In the following, we will perform the computer simulation.

$$
\begin{aligned}
C\frac{dV}{dt} &= I_{ext} - \overline{g}_K n^4 (V - E_K) + \overline{g}_{Na} m^3 h (V - E_{Na}) + \overline{g}_l (V - E_l) \\
\frac{dn}{dt} &= K_t (A_n (1 - n) - B_n n) \\
\frac{dm}{dt} &= K_t (A_m (1 - m) - B_m m) \\
\frac{dh}{dt} &= K_t (A_h (1 - h) - B_h h) \\
I_{ext} &= I_{offset} + I_{sig}
\end{aligned}
\tag{2}
$$

here, I_{sig} is the input signal.

$$K_t = 3^{(T-6.3)/10}$$

$$V' = V - V_{rest}$$

$$A_n = \frac{0.01*(10-V')}{e^{(10-V')/10}-1}$$

$$B_n = 0.125 * e^{(-V'/80)}$$

$$A_m = \frac{0.1*(25-V')}{e^{(25-V')/10}-1}$$

$$B_m = 4 * e^{(-V'/18)}$$

$$A_h = 0.07 * e^{-V'/20}$$

$$B_h = \frac{1}{e^{(30-V')/10}+1}$$

During the computing, the function parameters are shown as follows

Table 1.

Parameter	Default Value	Unit
C	1	uF cm-2
$\overline{g}_K$	36	mS cm-2
$\overline{g}_{Na}$	120	mS cm-2
$\overline{g}_l$	0.3	mS cm-2
E_K	-71.967	mv
E_{Na}	54.98	mv
E_l	-49	mv
I_{offset}	0	mA cm-2
T	6.3	°C
V_{rest}	-59.805	mv

Practically, when performing computer simulation the input signal is kind of periodic square wave, with its amplitude of 20mA/cm^2 and width of 1ms.

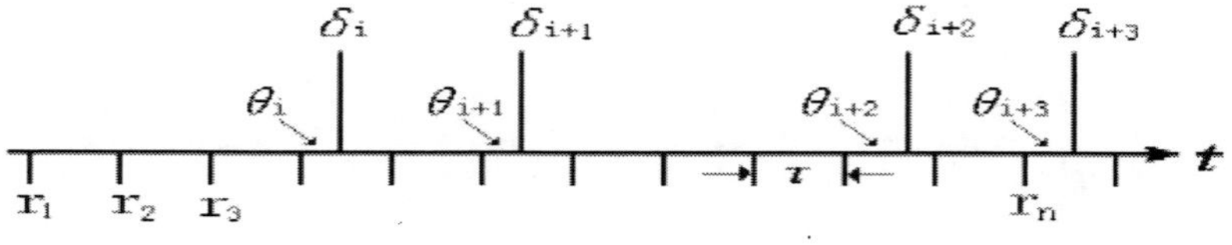

Figure 1. Circle mapping,δi is the output of neuron. ri is the input impulse (stimulation), serving as time scale.

The width selection of input signal is based on the typical width of action potential in real neural system. The numerical solution to H-H model is obtained by using Runge-Kutte method of variable step length. Practically, ode45, one of Matlab's routines is utilized with relative error of 1e-6, and absolute error of 1e-9. In calculation of variable step length, the minimum of the time step length ranges between 1e-8 and 1e-7, while the maximum between 0.01 and 0.1.

If the time when action potential reaches its peak is defined as the time point of the action potential, and the interval between the time point and the nearest previous time point is defined as impulse period, then impulse period of the neuron response changes irregularly, as shown in figure 1. Apply circle mapping to output signal [9, 10]. In detail, as shown in figure 1, draw the input periodic signal r_i as time scale, and, using the method illustrated in figure 1a, get the phase signals, such as $\theta_{i+1}\theta_{i+2}\theta_{i+3}......\theta_n$. This is the process how circle mapping is performed.

We have sequence:

$$\{\theta_i\} = \theta_1\theta_2\theta_3...\theta_n \tag{3}$$

(θ_i takes relative value)According to sequence (3), we can find the relationship as follows:

$$\theta_{n+1} = \Phi\ (\theta_n) \tag{4}$$

From the computer simulation, it can be seen that when a neural impulse sequence with equal interval (stimuli) is fed to one neuron (see figure 1), an impulse sequence with irregular period comes out, as shown in figure 1.

Because there is no explicit function expression, we can't get the concrete function for Φ. But we can draw its curve based on sequence (3). (See figure 2)

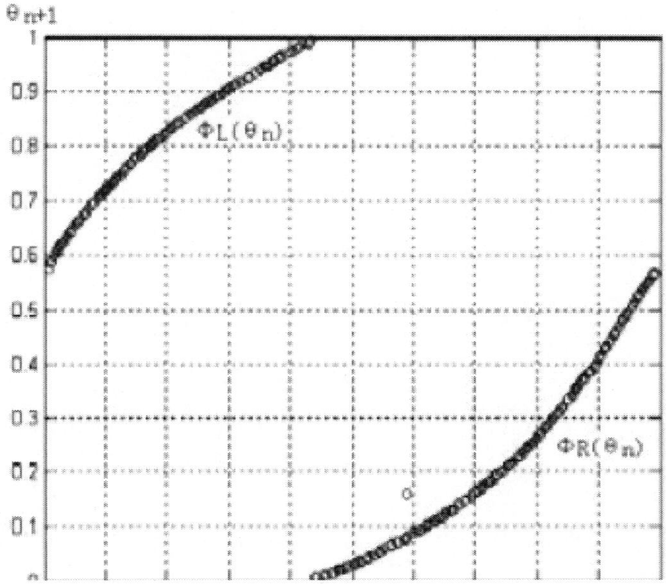

Figure 2. Circle mapping of neuron's output when the period of input impulse equals 2.6ms. Relative coordinate $\theta_i = \alpha_i/\tau$ is used ($\alpha_i \in (0,\tau)$),where r is the period of input signal (The isolated point is caused by our failure to handle the initial problem properly).

It is obviously that function between θ_n andθ_{n+1} is quite characteristic.

From the viewpoint of circle mapping theory, it is a monotonic increasing mapping. When we have an initial phaseθ_1, we can determineθ_2 according to figure 2. Continue in the similar way, a phase sequence can be obtained. This rule provides a solid base for us to understand neural coding. Next, we just begin to analyze this impulse sequence based on the rule of circle mapping.

3. Symbolic Dynamics for Circle Mapping

We will prepare to answer the second question: how trains of impulses can be ordered, which depends on symbolic dynamics method.

For it is a monotonic mapping above, According to [9, 10], this mapping is a monotonic increasing function, thus the creation and ordering regularity of this symbolic sequence will be relatively simple.

Suppose an output impulse sequence of neuron:

Assume that:

$$\eta = \delta_0, \delta_1, \delta_2, \ldots \delta_i, . \tag{5}$$

In the calculation, the period which impulse δ_{i-1} is in is used as the first period.

$$S_i = \begin{cases} p_1 & when\ \delta_i\ is\ in\ period\ 1 \\ p_2 & when\ \delta_i\ is\ in\ period\ 2 \\ p_3 & when\ \delta_i\ is\ in\ period\ 3 \\ & \cdots \\ p_r & when\ \delta_i\ is\ in\ period\ r \end{cases} \tag{6}$$

In the above equation, the period in which spike δ_{i-1} occurs is used as period 1.

According to (6), we can transform the impulse sequence $\eta=\delta_0\delta_1\delta_2\ldots\ldots\delta_i\ldots$ into a symbolic sequence.

$$\{s_i\} = s_1, s_2, s_3, \ldots\ldots, s_i, . \tag{7}$$

where $S_i = p_1, p_2, p_3, \ldots\ldots p_r$.

For example, in figure 1(a), impulses are transformed to symbols as:

$\delta_{i+1}(t) \rightarrow p_3$; $\delta_{i+2}(t) \rightarrow p_5$; $\delta_{i+3}(t) \rightarrow p_3$;

A impulse with initial phase θ_1 can determine an impulse sequence, and each impulse sequence will correspond to a symbolic sequence $\{S_i\}$.

Each symbolic sequence can be ordered by initial phase θ_1. The applied rule is:

On the assumption that there are two symbolic sequences:

$a_1a_2a_3\ldots\ldots a_n$ and $b_1b_2b_3\ldots\ldots b_n$

where, a_i and $b_1 = p_1, p_2, \ p_3, \ \text{----}, p_r$

Compare the first symbols of these two symbolic sequences, a_1 and b_1.

It is obvious that

$$p_1 < p_2 < p_3 \cdots p_i < \ldots < p_r \tag{8}$$

For symbolic sequences more than two, we have:

Here, $\Sigma = a_1a_2a_3\ldots\ldots a_i = b_1b_2b_3\ldots\ldots b_i$ represents the section of which the beginning i-bits of sequence are the same.

$$\sum p_1 < \sum p_2 < \ldots < \sum p_r \tag{9}$$

We don't need to know the values of all the initial phasesθ_1 .If the corresponding symbolic sequence of each initial phase is obtained, we can decide which value ofθ_1 is bigger. This is the rule of ordering by initial phase applied in symbolic dynamics.

4. The Ordering Rule for Response of Neurons Stimulated by Impulses of Different Frequencies

The ordering rule in (6) represents the ordering rule of initial phases. With the increasing of initial phaseθ_1, the mapping sequence increases also. Now we have a question: When the frequency of input impulse changes, will the output symbolic sequence be ordered with frequency? From the circle mapping theory, this is a problem concerning parameter ordering.

Suppose that all parameters remain unchanged in equation (2) as well as the initial value. Only the frequency (period τ) of the input impulse is changed.

From the curves in figure 3, we can see that circle mapping function curve moves towards low-right with the increasing of stimulation period τ. The right branch curve in the square of figure 3 will be replaced by the left branch, and at the same time a new branch will appear.

Note that there are some points in the panel with period value τ=2.4ms, It is mainly due to the drawing problem. First, we draw a long curve as figure 1.

Depending on its ergodicity, we draw most of the panels in figure 3. When the period becomes 2.4ms, periodic solution appears, resulting in only several points left. So it is with other figures.

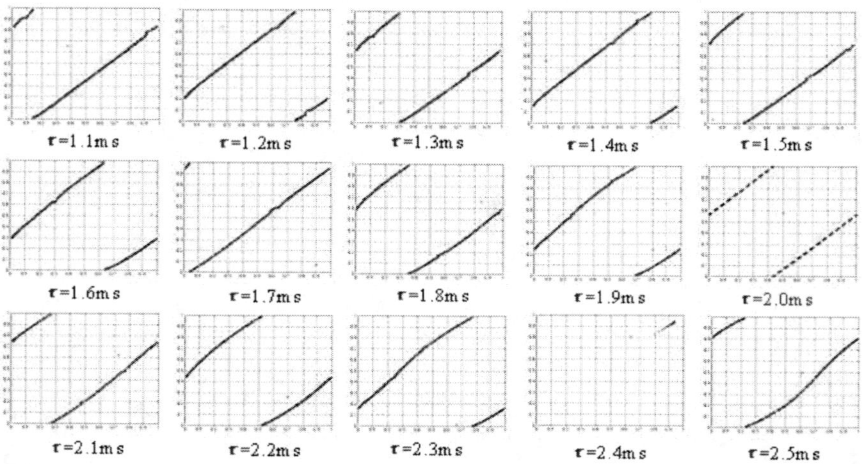

Figure 3. Function curve charge with the increasing of τ.

This mapping can be expressed with symbolic sequence, and symbol can be generated according to the equation (6). Let

$$\{a_i\} = a_1 a_2 a_3 \ldots\ldots a_i \ldots\ldots \tag{10}$$

$$a_i = p_1, p_2, p_3, \ldots, \ldots, p_r \tag{11}$$

here

$$i = 1, 2, 3, \ldots, n \tag{12}$$

In our discussion, let r=7 and P_i=i, we have Table 2. It appears three symbols in this table2.

Table 2.

Stimulated cycle (ms)	Another symbolic Sequence (20bits)
2.3	76666766667666766667
2.32	67666667666667666667
2.34	67666666667666666667
2.36	66766666666666666676
2.38	66667666666666666666
2.4	66666666666666666666
2.42	66666666666666665666
2.44	66666665666666666566
2.46	66665666666566666656
2.48	66656666566666566665
2.5	66566665666566656666

From Table 2, we can see that both period and output symbol are ordered. It also means that when input impulses with different frequencies stimulate the neuron, we can determine their frequencies by the output symbolic sequences.

5. Rules of Changes of Neuron with Respect to Ionic Channel and Other Parameters

Besides the change regularity of frequency parameter, we discover the similar change rules of other parameters.

5.1. Change of K Ionic Channel

Stimulus I_{sig} serves as input signal with cycle of 2.6ms, amplitude of 20mA cm^{-2}, the width of 1ms, and other conditions remaining the same as in figure 3 except that Only K^+ channel changes.

The maximal conductance $\overline{g}_K$ of K^+ channel varies in the range from 25 to 44mS cm^{-2}. See figure 4.

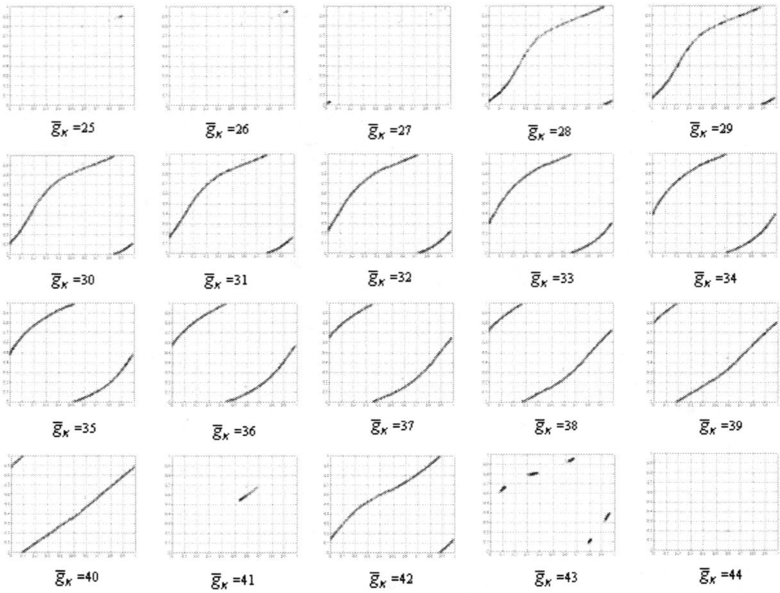

Figure 4. Function curves varies with k channel.

5.2. Change of Cell Membrane Capacitance

The condition remains the same except for membrane capacitance C. C changes in the range from 0.5 to 1.9 uF cm^{-2} with step of 0.1 uF cm^{-2}. The results are illustrated in the following in figure 5

5.3. Change of Na Ionic Channel

The conditions remain the same except for Na+ channel. The maximal conductance of Na+ channel changes in the range from 110 to 130mS cm^{-2}, as shown in figure 6. If the regularity of frequency change makes it possible to formulate the one-to-one correspondence between frequency and neural impulse sequence, then the regularity implied in figure 4.5.6 can be used to build correspondence between parameters of neurons and neural impulse sequences. Similarly, correspondences between physical quantity as well as chemical quantity, which will influence parameters of neuron, and neural impulse sequences can be formulated. Furthermore, frequency is used as an example in the following discussion.

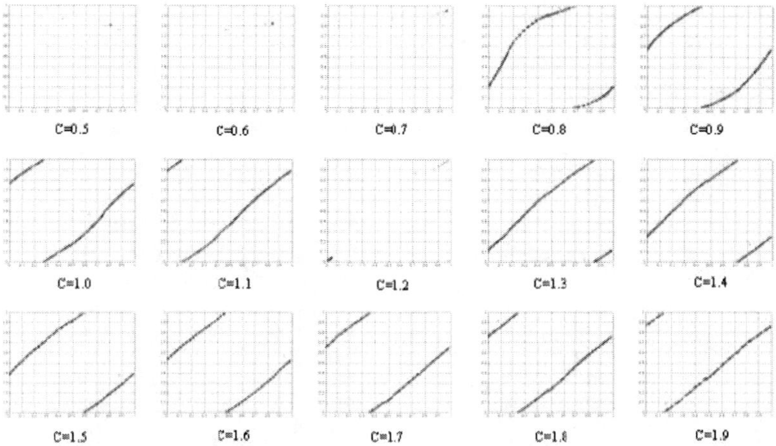

Figure 5. Function curves varies with capacitance C.

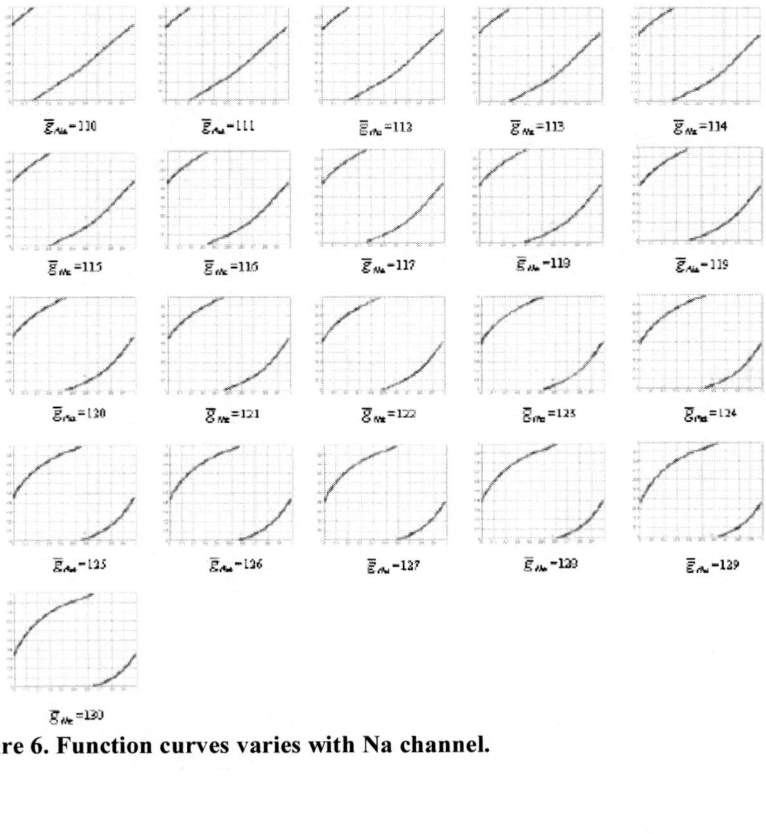

Figure 6. Function curves varies with Na channel.

6. Further Discussion on Circle Mapping

In figure 5, the circle mapping is very perfect. However, when the period gets longer, one segment of the left branch tends to be horizontal, just like the phenomena happening in figure 7, which indicates the critical end of monotonicity.

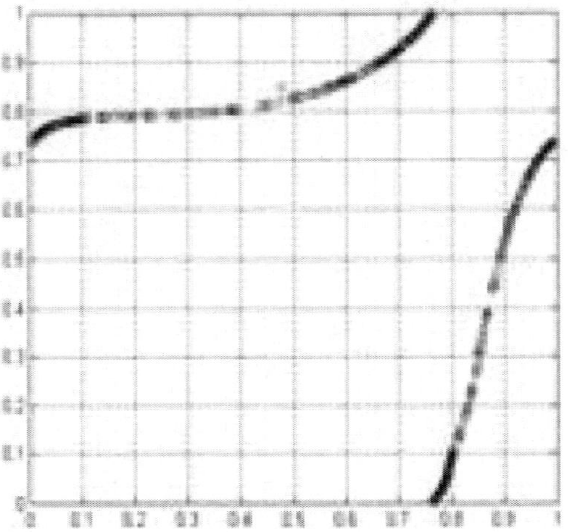

Figure 7. Period τ=3. 2.

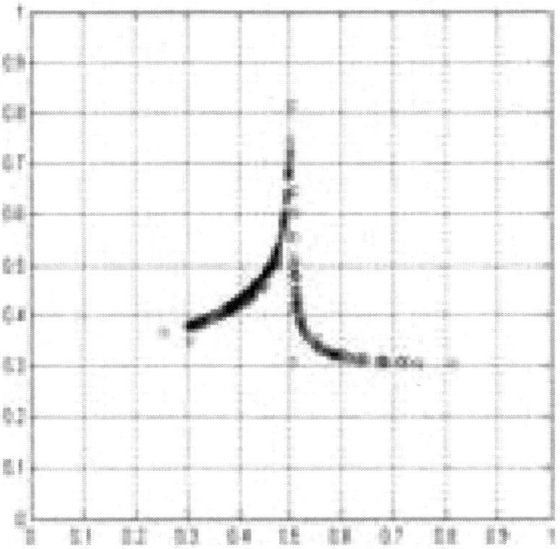

Figure 8. Period τ=6.

If the period is doubled again, the monotonicity rule of circle mapping changes in figure 8. We don't know whether it still has meanings for information processing.

What we can judge is that from the viewpoint of frequency testing, neuron has its own applicable range. Because of different parameters, the applicable frequency range for every neuron differs.

Experts of non-linear field favor especially complicated dynamic system, in particularly, the ones including many fixed points, limit cycle and bifurcations etc. However, some requirements have to be met before input signals can be ordered by impulse sequence. At least for the neural system, neither stable fixed point nor limit cycle is allowed to occur within the ordering scope of parameters (or initial value). If limit cycle does exist in the system, all orbits (impulse sequences) enter the limit cycle. All orbits superpose themselves together, which makes ordering impossible. From another viewpoint, can we draw the conclusion that if the impulse sequence can be ordered, neural system can't be working at the stable fixed point or stable limit cycle.

7. Signal Space, Orbit Space and Symbolic Space

All input signals of different frequencies are combined to constitute a signal space I. Every element $i_i\ (t)$ in signal space I is an impulse sequence of specific frequency, where t is a time variable.

Every input signal maps to an output orbit (impulse sequence) of neuron o_i. And all of these orbits constitute orbit space O (impulse sequence space O).

$$o_i \in O \quad i = 1,2,3,\ldots\ldots,n \tag{13}$$

$$o_i = o_i(t) \tag{14}$$

The mapping from I space to O space is

$$\Psi: \qquad I \to 0 \tag{15}$$

which is one-to-one. In this article, we have established the mapping between frequency signal and neural impulse sequence.

Every orbit can be transformed to a symbolic sequence according to equation (6). All the symbolic sequences s_i is formed a Symbolic Space *S*.

$$s_i \in S \tag{16}$$

The mapping from *O* space to *S* space is:

$$\Phi : \qquad O \to S \tag{17}$$

which is also one-to-one.

Now let's give distance definition.

Suppose two symbolic sequences,

$$A = \{a_i\} = a_1 a_2 a_3 a_4 \ldots a_i \ldots$$

$$a_i = p_1, p_2, p_3, \ldots, p_i, \ldots, p_r \tag{18}$$

$$B = \{b_i\} = b_1 b_2 b_3 b_4 \ldots b_i \ldots$$

$$b_i = p_1, p_2, p_3, \ldots, p_i, \ldots, p_r \tag{19}$$

$$d(A,B) = \left| \sum_{i=1}^{\infty} \frac{(a_i - b_i)}{r^i} \right| \tag{20}$$

Definition: the distance between sequence *A* and sequence *B* is

Obviously, this definition satisfies the three conditions of distance definition. The introduction of distance definition into symbolic space implies that it is a distance space. For a distance space, operations become possible. So, the third question mentioned in Introduction is solved, and therefore the foundation for information processing is found. In neural system, information processing is carried out after the external signal is led to an symbolic space, which is a distance space and supports transformation and operation.

For other signals such as temperature and ionic channel, similar definition and analysis are applicable.

Because correspondence relationship has been built among the three spaces, information processing issue can be handled in symbolic space, so practically we can set H-H model aside. No matter whether some ionic channels have not been included for consideration, no matter what parameter precision standard we have adopted, or no mater what new improvements have been contributed to H-H model, our analysis will not be influenced, if H-H model reflects the process of electrophysiology in quality. Because every change in ionic channel of neuron will finally be reflected in the two curves shown in figure 2, symbol generation won't be influenced as well as our analysis result, if the monotonicity of two curves doesn't change. So with symbolic space, it can be declared that in spite of some errors in quantity, the analysis result will not be affected adversely only when the correctness of H-H model in quality is guaranteed.

From another viewpoint, the instability of neuron parameter will cause the instability of neural network. For symbolic space, once the above requirements are satisfied, the result of information processing will not change. Perhaps this is the best explanation for the uncertainty and instability question in neural system.

8. Discussion

Based on the analysis above, we have the following conclusions:

a. With the help of circle mapping, it is possible for us to set up the one-to-one correspondence relationship between signal space I, impulse sequence space O and symbolic space S (At least one-to-one relationship can be built between the sub spaces in these spaces.). Moreover, distance is defined in space S; operations can be applied in distance space. Similarly, generalized Poincaré mapping also has the characteristics mentioned above. All of these form the foundations for further research on neural information processing. Also the first and second critical problems have been partly solved.
b. Similar to automata theory, once the basic unit is known a complicated system can be constituted. Therefore, it is important to find the basic unit for information processing in brain. Though we don't know much about the whole structure of information processing

in brain, the smallest unit for neural impulse sequence transformation has been found. Also, we find some transformation rules of the smallest unit. It provides the foundation for information processing.

c. This article discusses the ordering rule of impulse sequences. Ordering by frequency will be referred to as frequency coding. For equation (2), ordering rules of other parameters can also be found, in other words, coding of one parameter. It means that in different situations, there are different ordering rules for neuron. These different ordering rules reflect different information. In neural system these different information are combined together so that neural system has many functions.
d. Because correspondence relationship has been built among the signal space, orbit space and symbolic spaces, information processing issue can be handled in symbolic space. It is very important. In our opinion, information processing and signal detection in neural system are carried out in symbolic space. The uncertainty and instability problems may be solved in symbolic space.

Conclusion

In this work, circle mapping together with symbolic dynamics method is used to solve the problems mentioned above. It forms a base for the research of neural impulse information coding.

In summary, from the perspective of the two points proposed at the beginning of this article, the impulse sequence (InterSpike Interval, ISI) is believed to be more suitable for neural information coding.

References

[1] Gilles Laurent. A Systems Perspective on Early Olfactory Coding, *Science,* 286 723-728, (1999).

[2] Kandel Eric R, Squire Larry R. Neuroscience: Breaking down Scientific Barriers to the Study of Brain and Mind, *Science,* Vol 290, Issue 5494, 1113-1120, (2000).

[3] Jean-Pierre R, Petr L, Patricia DV, Andre D. Spiking frequency versus odorant concentration in olfactory receptor neurons, *BioSystems,* 58:133-141, (2000).

[4] Lestienne R. Impulse timing, synchronization and information processing on the sensory side of the central nervous system. *Prog Neurobiol,* 65(6): 545-691, (2001).

[5] Lovejoy LP, Shepard PD, Canavier CC. Apamin-induced Irregular Firing in Vitro and Irregular Single-Spike Firing Observed in vivo in Dopamine Neurons is Chaotic, *Neuroscience,* Vol. 104, No. 3, pp. 829-840, (2001).

[6] Hoppensteadt Frank. Modeling the Cumulative Distribution Function of Impulses in *Neural Networks International Journal of Bifurcation and Chaos,* Vol. 14, No. 51549-1558, (2004).

[7] Averbeck BB, Lee D. Coding and transmission of information by neural ensembles. *Trends Neurosci,* 27(4): 225-230, 2004.

[8] Galizia C Giovanni, Menzel Randolf. The role of glomeruli in the neural representation of odours: Results from optical recording studies. *Journal of Insect Physiology*, 47 115-130, (2001).

[9] Kim S, Ostlund S. Universal scaling in circle maps. *Physica D,* 39 365-392(1989).

[10] Zhang Zhong-jian, Chen Shi-Gang. Symbolic Dynamics of The Circle Map, *Acta Physica Sinica.* 38(1) 1-8, (1989).

[11] Meunier Claude, Segev Idan. Playing the Devil's advocate: Is the Hodgkin-Huxley model useful. *Trends Neurosciences,* 25 No.11, (2002).

[12] Kensaku Mori, Hiroshi Nagao, Yoshihiro Yoshihara. The Olfactory Bulb: Coding and Processing of Odor Molecule Information, *Science,* 286 711-715, (1999).

[13] Magdalena S, Oliver S, Bacigalupo J. Excitation, inhibition, and suppression by odors in isolated toad and rat olfactory receptor neurons *Am J Physiol Cell Physiol,* 279: C31–C39, (2000).

[14] Kaplan Daniel T, Clay John R, Manning Timothy, Glass L, Guevara MR and Shrier A. Subthreshold Dynamics in Periodically Stimulated Squid Giant Axons. *Physical Rev Letters*, 76, No. 21 1074-1077, (1996).

Chapter 4

Cognitive Axioms as Low-Level Rules of Communicative and Other Practices in Social Dynamical Systems

Evguenia V. Liutikova*
Independent Researcher, Zhukovsky, Moscow Region, Russia

Abstract

Research data in basic social cognition forms - attitudes, beliefs, stereotypes, prejudices, social representations - provide for treating these mental foundations of social cognition and behaviour as having a common principal function of *cognitive axioms* in perceiving, interpreting, and applying information to social practises. Cognitive axioms are shared by sociomental groups (people similarly interpreting the information received: T. M. Dridze's term) and, being endowed with value status, can be observed to regulate and constrain human mental and practical activities, functioning as a set of order parameters (*axiomatic threshold* function) and low-level rules for automodelled human-environmental interactions. The individual complex of interactions connecting a human to environment, *conversion mode* (after J. Huxley's term for matter circulation in nature), can be viewed as an axioms-based and resulting from selectivity of an individual mind or a sociomental group in interacting with environmental elements as to induce a resonant arousal. Cognitive axioms also underlie the enactment of the basic mechanism in persuasive, suggestion-implying communication, which, according to the vast research in the field, works through recipients recognising 'self-evident' meanings in a message. The most uncontroversial recognition of cognitive axioms in the form of

* Corresponding Author's Email: liutikova_ev@mail.ru.

In: Neuroscience and Technology Transform the Educational Ecosystem
Editors: Franco F. Orsucci and Nicoletta Sala
ISBN: 979-8-88697-157-6

suggestion-implying textual elements could be enacted in the minds of an *optimal audience* - a modelled recipient group. Persuasive communication, or social suggestion processes can be considered as evolving in LS-regime, with a message functioning as nonequilibrium, far-from-equilibrium, and critically nonequilibrium, depending on vigour and aggression in the response of an audience. The second and third modes of nonequilibrium interpretation of a message can cause a kind of phase transition in a receiving mind, driving it over a certain *critical semantic threshold*, with the meanings perceived considerably energising the audience conversion modes and changing their properties. Transcending the threshold may be combined with *semantic resonance* - the negative resonant divergence in different sociomental groups interpreting the signs equally crucial for the conversions of the group members. The responses of a society to environmental challenges, depending upon the practised conversion modes and shared axioms, may generate such *societal communicative situations* as, e.g., communicative stability, communicative challenge, and communicative crisis, with possible outcomes for the latter including communicative revolution, communicative jump, communicative stylisation, and communicative isolation. Certain preexisting axioms and conversion modes may recur later in social history in case they match the reproduced environmental conditions evidently so as to form, or to approach to, topologically correct 'agent-environment' interactive structures.

Keywords: cognitive axioms, social dynamical systems, persuasive communication, optimal audience, semantic resonance, societal communicative situations

1. Introduction

According to the Maturana-Varela theory, human consciousness is not necessarily sealed from the outer influence or fixed in its processes. Still, there are, more often than not, certain boundaries to an external impact on human mind and limitations to its flexibility, which can vary in power across different social environments. Actually, we can say that these boundaries and limitations take rather well-known social cognitive forms, such as *prejudices, stereotypes, attitudes, beliefs, social representations*. These social cognitive forms are important contributors to communicative, cognitive, and decision-making processes (Simon 1967, Tversky and Kahneman 1973, Holsti 1977, Winograd 1977, Tajfel 1981, Kennamer 1989, Aronson 1995, Nolan et al. 1999).

More generally, the mental-behavioural phenomena that mostly pertain to subconscious and half-conscious domains of human mind, like (1) the a priori foundations of general perception (comprising the selective perception mechanism), (2) beliefs, attitudes, (3) self-concepts, the foundations of social perception and attribution, stereotypes, prejudices, implicit personality theories, (4) the a priori foundations of logic and reasoning, cognitive schemata, cognitive clichees, social representations, (5) individual and collective fears (phobias) and the elements of the collective unconscious, - all of these are self-evident in meaning for their agents and capable of working as axiomatic foundations of cognition, speech, and action - *cognitive axioms.* The axioms form a kind of a systemic complex in a human mind, as they all share, at least, one principal function and one principal characteristic: (A) Each of these mental forms can be activated to serve as the basis for a cognitive process, in acquiring some new knowledge, and to set a standard, a norm, or a value against which information coming to a particular consciousness can be assessed and evaluated. (B) These mental forms are shaped and transferred mostly in the course of persuasive communication, or social suggestion, and represented by the suggestive elements of messages. Suggestive element of a message should be 'recognised' and accepted by recipients as their own self-evident meaning, without any doubts or controversy, which could require drawing on to critical thinking (see e.g., John Locke in his 'An essay on human understanding,' and also Sherif et al. 1965: 222, Bettinghaus 1980, Cialdini 1988, Petty and Cacioppo 1981, Rokeach 1972:34-35, O'Donnell and Jowett 1989). A group of recipients that would be able to react uncontroversially to the cognitive axioms expressed or implied in a given text can be called *optimal audience* for the text (Lioutikova 2006). This concept is built on the idea of 'sociomental groups' comprising the people, across society, who 'similarly interpret textually organised information, due to the common values, attitudes, expectations, mentality, etc.' (Dridze 2000:29, 25, cf. 'interpretive societies' in Fish 1994(1980):188-190, 'different publics' in Moscovici 1985, and 'epistemic communities' in Jepperson et al. 1996). Certainly, the 'optimal audience' is primarily a theoretical concept, but in reality we can find different levels of approximation to this ideal model.

In their inactive state, cognitive axiomatic forms can be defined as *suggestive patterns.* Suggestive patterns with axiomatic functions are rather often traditional and shared by members of sociomental group (cf. Clark and Clark 1947, Lippman 1954, Rokeach 1972, Doise 1978, Moscovici 1993 - on the traditionality of different social cognitive forms). Which of the patterns will be assimilated/ internalised by an individual mind, eventually depends on an individual way of life and an acquired sense of what is real and natural or possible in the surrounding world. As Gareth Morgan put it, ‘culture gives us our world’ and ‘it traps us in that world’ (1997:229). Axiomatic suggestive patterns can be adopted in the process of education or can be derived from the preceding individual experience. In both cases, they act as lawful generalisations bearing on the further social activities. The suggestive patterns retain their axiomatic function until they continue making sense for a human and underlying some kind of activity within an individual way of life. Such patterns can assume different forms and be stored and then activated in human brain sometimes as words, sometimes as images or even ‘shadows’ of images.

Cognitive axioms as basic premises for perceiving and interpreting information both powerfully influence human-environmental interactions comprising an individual or a group lifestyle and are influenced by such lifestyle in a ‘feedback’ process: the structure of an axiomatic complex and the content of the axioms involved, in their turn, generally depend on the modes of individual or group interactions with environment.

We can regard human-environmental interactions as energy exchange processes bounded by human cognitive constraints - basic meanings in the form of cognitive axioms. The idea of knowledge-energy or information-energy relations is reflected in Otto Roessler’s schema which connects the positive-feedback processes for receiving energy to the processes of obtaining information through another positive-feedback relationship, as suggested in Roessler’s lecture on theoretical biology at the Max-Planck-Institute for Behavioural Physiology of Sea Organisms, in 1966. The quality of such human ‘mind-energy system’ should be determined by both common and individual information-energy needs which can be regarded as functionally expanded corollaries to the needs from the system suggested by the renown psychologist A. Maslow (see also Reymers 1994:304, 294) and are important contributors to developing a personal way of life and, in their turn, considerably influenced by it. The processes in a ‘mind-energy’ system are obviously dominated by two principal factors - genetics and socialisation of an individual. Thus, information-energy needs can be adopted through education or may even be inherited through genetic mechanisms (cf. Lumsden-Wilson theory of genetic and cultural coevolution (1981), see also H. Eysenck about genetically inherited human behavioural preferences for certain situations (1982:29)). As C. Langton aphoristically put it, ‘biological and cultural evolutions were simply two aspects of the same phenomenon, and <...> the “genes” of culture were beliefs - which in turn were recorded in the basic DNA of culture: language’ ((1978), see Waldrop 1993:214).

Information-energy needs can assume, in particular, the form of more or less conscious dependency on certain personal meanings which can guide the necessary interactions along the lines of 'energy affinity' and 'energy complementarity'. To become a valuable energiser for a given personal behavior, the developed or adopted meaning (sense) should provide for establishing a positive-feedback relation with environment, through a relevant interaction (cf. the concept of a rewarded social interaction formulated by the renowned sociologist G. K. Homans (1961)).

The system, embracing fundamental, personally energising meanings and their functions, in the form of human-environmental interactions, presents a personal way of energy exchange with environment, which is the most suitable, given the personal characteristics and the environmental circumstances, for a given human's survival and self-actualisation. Such system can be named *'conversion,'* on the analogy of the term, suggested by the renowned British biologist, Julian Huxley, for the energy and matter cycle in nature (1961:30). Put another way, the conversion in question is a complex of multilevel energy exchange processes, relating persons to different aspects of their environment.

Within a society sharing some common cultural grounds, individual conversions are sure to display typical traits. Individual conversions of the same type must reveal the identical hierarchical patterns of the leading and secondary energy exchange processes within their frameworks, i.e., the same relative significance of these processes for a particular conversion type.

2. Axiomatic Foundations of Cognition and Communication from the Dynamical Systems' Perspective

H. N. Knyazeva and S. P. Kurdyumov suggest the view of a human consciousness as 'a complex, hierarchical organisation, incorporating the levels with different amount of chaotic structures and different tempo-worlds' (2002:230). Elaborating on the details of the organisation's functioning, these authors hypothesise 'a certain potentially distinguished, dominating direction of developments,' which organises the system of neural networks against the background of 'marked nonlinearity' and 'determined chaos' (Knyazeva and Kurdyumov 2002:195,196, see also Basar et al. 1983, Dreymanis 1987, Farmer 1982:243, Haken 1984:2). Grounding on these assumptions, partly hypothesised and partly experimentally supported, it is possible to venture another hypothesis: a cognitive axiom may present a certain 'dominating' contour of a given neural network's activation, which arises due to certain rules, underlying the organisation of this network, and is so deeply rooted in the functional properties of individual consciousness and the constituting properties of individual organism, as to be reproduced (fully or partly, depending on circumstances) in individual activities - interactions with environment. The definition suggested is rather close to the definition of mental schemas, formulated by R. D. Stacey, where schema is viewed as 'a pattern of electrical activity' passing through synapses between neurons and 'modeling a particular regularity in the mass of stimuli confronting a brain at any one time' (1996:37). Thus, cognitive axiomatics may be regarded as low-level rules, determining the state of a complex system - individual consciousness. The activation of axioms may be described in terms of an automodelled process, with the axioms as a basis for automodelled interactions within the framework of individual conversion (cf. R. D. Stacey on the limits of efficiency in work of operational schemas (1996:90). Then, suggestive patterns with latent axiomatic functions may be treated as such contours of neural networks' activation that, though easily switched on within human consciousness, are not presently influential in the human's activities (cf. R. D. Stacey on recessive schemas (1996:135)).

The limiting function of axiomatics can be modelled in the concept of *axiomatic threshold*, which can be defined as periodical interpretation-regulating function of an adopted axiomatic complex, which sets (1) the limits of plausibility for interpreting the coming information, (2) the limits of feasibility for a given person interacting with environment, (3) the limits and determinations for an aggregate of personal meanings (personal semantics), basic for a given way of life. This is basically fits in with Maturana-Varela theory, according to which living systems, being self-referential, 'cannot enter into interactions that are not specified in the pattern of relations that define their organization' and, therefore, 'a system's interaction with its "environment" is really a reflection and a part of its own organization" (see Morgan 1997:253-254). It can be said that the concept of axiomatic threshold, in a sense, adds to the psychological concept of sensory threshold, and is essentially close to the idea of constructive alternativism (Kelly 1955:21) and the idea of 'broad' and 'narrow' cognitive limitations (Dunn 1994). The limits imposed by an axiomatic threshold on a given consciousness follow the limitations of the 'semantic field' produced by an axiomatic complex which is adopted by the consciousness. This total 'semantic field' of cognitive axiomatics is shaped by the aggregate of minor 'semantic fields' resulting from separate axioms in a complex.

Normally, people are unconscious of the axiomatic threshold functioning, but in a critical situation they may become suddenly aware of the limits it imposes on their minds and activities. That is why, in my opinion, the threshold should be defined as a periodical function of axiomatic semantic field. Axiomatic threshold can be viewed as boundary (or marginal) constraints for building the arousal contours within a neural network. Given the neural network's properties of self-organisation and self-evolution, pertaining to it as a living system, such boundary constraints can change, which may lead to increasing complexity (metaphorically speaking, to 'the raising of axiomatic threshold'), decreasing complexity ('the lowering of axiomatic threshold'), expanding the structure through activating latent capabilities or contracting the structure through switching off the actual functions allowed by the existing boundary constraints (an axiomatic threshold 'shifting on the same plane'). The dynamics of axiomatic threshold and suggestive patterns with potential axiomatic function can be viewed as the sources of potential increase in complexity of human mind and behaviour. Axiomatic threshold's flexibility is more effective when an axiomatic set is on the verge of chaos - i.e., in critical situations.

3. The Way of Life Viewed as a Dynamical Structure: The Concept of Conversion

As determined above, conversion is a dynamical representation of a way of life seen as a complex of multilevel energy exchange processes, relating an individual to different aspects of environment. A conversion profile can be viewed as resulting from selectivity of an individual mind or a sociomental group in interacting with environmental elements as to induce a resonant arousal. Each conversion mode can experience a topologically correct resonant arousal, manifesting the mode's efficiency and 'success,' only through a contact with specifically relevant energisers within environment, the selection being determined by the most important personal meanings (axioms) and the information-energy needs, pertaining to a concrete conversion. The topologically correct conversion organisation evidently can provide for the more rapid evolution and, thus, for the higher tonicity in certain types or sets of interactions. Weak fluctuations within conversion, which may include random thoughts as random arousal contours in neural networks or random, singularly performed interactions with environment, normally will not overcome the sensitivity barrier, but beyond this barrier - e.g., in a critical life situation, - their impact can be considerably amplified.

The optimal combination of a concrete conversion mode or type with the time and place of its enactment may set a kind of behavioural model in certain sociohistoric conditions. Given the correct resonance with favourable environment and the information-energy needs of other people, a certain conversion mode can rise from ‘a private affair’ through a sociomental group mode to the larger society conversion attractor.

4. Suggestiveness Actualising as Suggestion: The Contributors to the Process

As the messages, both deliberately constructed for suggestive perception and one-hundred per cent effective in performing the task, present, in fact, a very specific case in communication, here we are dealing primarily with suggestive textual elements, resulting rather from the nature of a message source than from a deliberate calculation of a communicator and permeating a great amount of texts on various subjects.

The suggestive elements of a message here refer to the elements, potentially capable of activating everyday axiomatic meanings in audience minds. For the needs of research in these elements, in my opinion, it is useful to distinguish between *suggestiveness*, as *a message quality*, and *suggestion*, as *an actual message’s function,* which is enacted by the perceiving minds of real audience.

The ability to consciously manipulate suggestive elements within a message on a given subject can be unequally distributed among members of some social hierarchy - in accordance with the members’ relations to the process of generating and controlling suggestive meanings with axiomatic potential. Thus, on the top of this scale we find an ‘absolute’ manipulator (the term here refers to a person striving to persuade an audience of something that correlates with these people’s goals, but not with their beliefs (cf. the renowned French social psychologist S. Moscovici about ‘fanatic’ and a person of belief (1985)), and at the bottom we find an ‘absolute’ suggestor (the term here refers to a person striving to impose his own beliefs upon audience). Generally, almost anyone of us is somehow susceptible to different kinds of social suggestion and somehow inclined to use it in our communicative practices.

4.1. The Conversion Characteristics

Though suggestive perception may occur almost within any conversion complex, some people are markedly more susceptible to suggestion-implying information. A conversion mode pertaining to such people should obviously show:

1. *The high isolation level,* featuring considerably limited interactions between a conversion agent and environment, the agent being heavily dependent on very few energy sources. Consequently, such person may lack a habit of verifying the information received and, at the same time, be denied the access to the social and information resources necessary to accomplish such verification. The interpretation strategies of such persons, based on their interpretation capacities, are likely to converge to a sort of simple linear algorithms.
2. *The high positive entropy level,* featuring the high energy consumption and inefficient energy feedback in the personal interactions with environment. For instance, such person may experience fatigue for quite a long period of time, and the suggestive mode of interpreting the information received partly allows this agent 'to spare the efforts'.
3. *The high linearity level,* in the organisation of conversion elements, featuring the rigidly structured contact between an agent and environment. Such constraints may arise due to the peculiarities of individual consciousness as well as due to the properties of a social context incorporating individual activities (e.g., in totalitarian society). In the former case, the image of environment within individual mind is very likely to have markedly hierarchical structure, the individual tending to obey authorities. A person, internally motivated to obey, is obviously more inclined to suggestive perception of the information received from the acknowledged authorities. In the 'totalitarian' case, obviously, the obedience to authorities may be externally motivated, with suggestive perception outwardly expressed, but not always internally adopted.

4. *The high monotony level,* in the rhythm of conversion processes, featuring aggressive interactions between the conversion agent and related environment, or considerable aggressive potential within the framework of a given conversion (e.g., due to the high entropy level). Such enmity pertaining to the relations between a human and environment can provoke a sudden and sharp increase in energy consumption within the human's conversion and further promote selectivity in conversion interactions (and thus increasing its isolation), while driving the interactions to a more rigid structure (and thus enhancing the linearity of conversion). Thus, high monotony level in a conversion should almost invariably provide for the conditions rather favourable for 'switching on' entropy growth. Therefore, high monotony in conversion may not only be generated by high entropy potential but, in its turn, generate it. Consequently, it may be said that high monotony in conversion leads to high susceptibility to suggestion-implying communication. The suggested conversion characteristics are essentially close to three control parameters for complex adaptive systems as marked out by R. D. Stacey (1996:99).

4.2. The Contributing Properties of Communicative Culture within a Sociomental Group

Listed below are the communicative cultural factors in a sociomental group, featured in certain typical characteristics of the group conversion parameters that act on suggestiveness actualising in suggestion:

1. The less isolated conversion modes in a given sociomental group, the wider their range of possible interactions with environment and, consequently, the more numerous the alternative sources of information available for the group members.
2. The higher the nonlinearity level within the conversion frameworks in a sociomental group, the more flexible the group members' strategy of interpreting the messages received, the less rigid their application of axiomatics in the course of such interpretation. It should be noted here that one of minor characteristics featuring the rigidity level (combining the qualities of isolation and linearity) of a given axiomatic complex is imagination capacity (cf. the special US

Congress committee report mentioning the lack of imagination among the important reasons of drawbacks in US special services' work shortly before 11 September, 2001 (Final Report 2004).

3. The lower the entropy level displayed by conversion modes of a sociomental group, the more active the group members interpreting in case any message is received. It should be marked, however, that the low entropy combined with the highly influential axiomatics and highly monotonic conversion mode, in case certain information is suggestively perceived, may lead to aggressive social activities of the group members, with their interpretive activities simultaneously being quite low. Deviant youth groups may provide an example of such behaviour.
4. The less monotonic the interactions within the conversion frameworks in a given sociomental group, the more tolerant the attitudes of the group members to alternative interpretations of the information coming.

5. Dynamical Systemic Approach in Analysing the Messages with Suggestive Elements

Considered in this paragraph are several and, in my view, most important features of suggestion-implying communication, regarded from the dynamical systems' perspective. To start with, it is possible to speak about nonequilibrium in suggestion-implying messages, with the following grades:

1. *Nonequilibrium text* - a message, which suggestive elements promote a change in the attitude of a target audience toward a certain subject or event.
2. *Far-from-equilibrium text* - a message, which suggestive elements inspire a target audience to act in regard to such environmental aspect that hitherto, in their eyes, did not require any active treatment.
3. *Critically nonequilibrium text* - a message, which suggestive elements can stimulate a target audience to an aggressive action where the audience hitherto did not mean to act in such way (cf. phase 5, destruction, of negating behavior in Allport, 1954).

The probability of a communicative system's transition to a nonequilibrium state depends on whether an audience will recognise its significant axiomatic meanings in the suggestive elements of a message and whether the message will be perceived as informing of a certain threat to such significant meanings. Generally, the more significant aspects in the relations of an audience with the world are organised, within the audience minds, as suggestive patterns with axiomatic function, the more ready the audience to receive different kinds of nonequilibrium messages. It is quite possible that some conversion processes, pertaining to such people, will be characterised by enhanced isolation and monotony and, consequently, enhanced potential aggressiveness. If there are no data which characterise an actual audience's perception of a certain message as a suggestive nonequilibrium communicative process, the message can only be qualified as a potentially nonequilibrium. The potential nonequilibrium quality, in my view, is induced by the following factors:

1. The power of, and the relationships between, connotations within the text.
2. The trajectory of a text logic.
3. The presence of semes that can cause fear for, or inform of a threat to, axiomatic meanings important for a target audience.
4. The presence of the components of an 'alien' archetype (is often combined with factor (3)).
5. The representation of message meanings through two or more alternative viewpoints, implying juxtaposition of alternative values and expressed in related opposing connotations. This results in emergence of peculiar suggestive 'bifurcation points' within a text, provoking a recipient to choose between the viewpoints of communicators and their opponents and, consequently, to choose between the different modes of interpreting the whole message. In such case, the organisation of suggestive elements within a text can guide the recipients' interpretation along the line, most suitable for suggestion-implying communication, thus compromising the 'free-choice' situation.
6. The presence of referents to some powerful factors in the extralinguistic (social) context of message, which can guide interpretation process in a target audience (e.g., appeal to a social or ideological authority or opinion leader). Such referents are more frequent at suggestive 'bifurcation points' in a message.

7. Such mode of interpreting sociohistoric experience, adopted by a given culture, that promotes social suggestion of a nonequilibrium quality, - as is often the case with historic myths.

The relative efficiency of the factors listed depends on significance, for a given audience, of the suggestive patterns activated, and on the social context of their activation. Nonequilibrium activation of suggestive patterns with axiomatic functions may result from a single message or a series of messages on the same subject, received by audience at different time intervals. In the latter case, the nonequilibrium rate can increase from message to message, as it goes, for example, with texts, composed by experienced manipulators and meant for 'warming' an audience up to a required state. But that is also the way suggestors act if a certain factor continuously increase the nonequilibrium rate in their interactions with environment.

If the same sociomental group repeatedly receives and interprets verbal pieces of information where message purposes are similar and principal statements are close in meaning, the resulting picture of such situations may be presented as a Cantor set featuring the diachronic signature of communicative semantic dynamics across consecutive communication processes involving a given sociomental group (cf. J. A. Berger and C. Heath on the habitat and fluctuation of ideas (2005)). The trajectory, generating a Cantor set on a plane, thus will represent the cycle of the given meanings circulating across the other segments of society and recurring to the interpreting sociomental group as updated information on the same subject. The set of points - intermediately related meanings, forming the attractor, will feature a set of possible interpretations for the information recurring. Therefore, the structure of a semantic attractor, revealed by the information circulation, will present probabilistic model of evolution in the interpretation of a coherent semantic complex by a certain sociomental group. The total amount of information, as being comprehended and accumulated by the group, may be considered as infinitely increasing parameter. The character of a trajectory and period of intersecting with the plane of semantic attractor will depend on the properties, 'repertoire,' and periods in the interactions of a given group with environment. Minds, comprised in a sociomental group, will act as selectors within information flow. The smaller the cycle of a trajectory and the more the group minds are inclined to select messages close in meaning, the higher the risk of these minds' transition to a far-from-equilibrium or critically nonequilibrium state, in regard to the suggestive meanings received.

A single text may also function as a semantic attractor if it is popular and influential within a given culture, with its principal meanings, as extracted by an interpreting audience, being identical or similar to the conversion-regulating meanings adopted by the audience minds. The time of a text serving as an attractor will depend on duration of such semantic similarity state. Semantic sets, more or less persistent within a certain culture, - e.g., in the form of ideology or mythology, - can work as attractors as well.

Depending on a manipulator's goal or a suggestor's disposition, the set of suggestive elements in a message may (a) appeal to the axiomatics as adopted by the audience and correlating with a target semantic attractor, (b) tend to 'reorient' the axiomatics of audience toward another target semantic attractor already existing, (c) tend to set a new semantic attractor, with reorienting the axiomatics of audience toward it.

Far-from-equilibrium and critically nonequilibrium interpretations of suggestive elements in a message may be regarded as a kind of 'phase transition' in a state of the minds in audience and are marked with transcending certain *critical semantic thresholds*, beyond which the meanings received may considerably energise the audience conversion modes and change the properties of related interactions with environment. This correlates with sensitivity threshold in complex systems, beyond which an impact effect for them is strongly amplified. Socially, this can correspond to new interpretation of environmental developments, rapidly and massively spread within a societal space, due to e.g., propagandist effect in a critical social situation. Thus, a far-from-equilibrium impact of suggestive text on a given audience can be explained by nonlinear positive feedback operating in every point of a societal space - in every receiving mind. Such recipients experience a sort of resonant disturbance while interpreting suggestive elements of the message received - when they recognise the elements' meanings as similar or identical to their own axiomatics. Resulting from such spatial positive feedback, which integrates multiple moments of recipients recognising the meanings received, a 'superfast evolution' of the communicative situation may be induced - i.e., the change of audience behaviour to the mode, defined by semantic attractor featured in a message.

Transcending a critical semantic threshold may be combined with negative *semantic resonance* emerging. The negative semantic resonance can be defined as a resonant divergence in different sociomental groups interpreting the signs equally crucial for the group members conversion modes (cf. the process labelled by P. Ricoeur as the conflict of interpretations (1974)). The meanings thus obtained stimulate different (sometimes 'diametrically' opposed in their orientation) social activities in the groups. This can lead to the situation when at least two sociomental groups are competing for 'the only true' (that is, essentially suggestive) interpretation of a given seme or semantic set.

Therefore, in communicative systems the nonequilibrium may emerge as a state of minds within a certain sociomental group, caused by specifically interpreting some part of semantics in a given message. Such nonequilibrium state of mind then may be transferred to the level of conversion practises. Given the knowledge about such practises in the different sociomental groups, relevant domains of potentially nonequilibrium semes/ meanings could be identified. The interpretation of such semes, by a sociomental group under study, is capable of increasing the risk of nonequilibrium activation of meanings and, consequently, the risk of nonequilibrium transition, for the conversion modes within the group.

6. Societal Communicative Situations Seen through Human Conversion Activity and Axiomatic Functioning

The last section of this article is focused on the communicative aspects of societal environmental challenges and human responses. Basic premises for this section are:

a. On a societal scale, a current environmental situation (including environmental challenge if any) is produced, in particular, by integrated human conversion activities preceding as well as simultaneous to the situation in question.
b. Society's response to an environmental challenge depends upon the quality of most influential and active minds (basically, upon the quality of cognitive axioms that constrain and guide their thinking and practical activities).
c. The nature of information diffusion processes within a society generally favours the emerging of fractal patterns at different levels of the 'individual - society' system.
d. Humans are living self-conscious dynamical systems, able to regulate and improve their interactions with environment through comprehending the information obtained in the course of these

interactions and, consequently, able to autonomously regulate the level of their openness and isolation.

e. There can be specific individual conversion modes, relatively autonomous from, and actually nonintegrable with, the majority of other human conversions within the society, which can be regarded as locales displaying steady autonomous dynamics in a societal dynamical system. In a model reflecting the general picture of conversion modes functioning in a society, these can be presented as power conversion points.

6.1. Sme Typical Communicative Situations in Dynamical Social Systems

Across different sociohistoric contexts, it is possible to single out a few, rather common types of societal communicative situations:

6.1.1. Communicative Stability

This type of situation is characterised by multiple, dynamically steady states of different sociomental groups within a larger society in quasistationary state. In a pluralistic, 'ideologically nonlinear' society such communicative regime prevails until minor social systems manage to maintain metastability and a relatively synchronised tempo rate through sequential stages in their changing. It is allowed by balanced combination of change and conservatism in the evolution of axiomatics and conversion modes within social subsystems (subcultures), with essentially the same attractors - in the forms of axiomatic and conversion structures - conserved throughout a stable period. This leads to energetically balanced nature of group-environmental activities and between-group interactions. Under the conditions, any disturbances, induced by inter- or in-group tensions and conflicts, should be local, short-ranged, and of weak amplitude and thus rather easy to overcome, for a social system with high nonlinearity properties.

Communicative stability is also markedly expressed in 'ideologically linear,' monotonous societies. But, possessing strong conservative properties, such systems, in the long run, are more vulnerable to societal disturbances.

6.1.2. Communicative Challenge

This imbalanced situation is characterised by a considerably hard collision between the cognitive axiomatics, adopted by a given sociomental group, with forcely and rapidly changed perception of the surrounding reality by the group members. As a result, the previously adopted axioms cease to function as 'order factors' that organise conversion modes and guide interactions within them. And previously latent mental structures, 'sleeping' suggestive patterns, emerge to perform axiomatic functions (cf. V. D. Nechayev on people in critical situations, turning to the cultural subconscious accumulated throughout the social history: 2002:16). If reshaping the existing axioms and conversion modes requires the amount of activation energy that places too hard a demand on resources of the agents involved, the situation may result in these agents' feeling the compensatingly increased need for suggestion-implying communication - as an energy or sedative resource. This may eventually lead to desadaptation, of various degrees, displayed by different sociomental groups or individuals in such society.

6.1.3. Communicative Crisis

This state arises from the long-time absence of effective solutions for the situation of communicative challenge. 'Long time' means the duration sufficient as to cause energy exhaustion of conversion agents involved in meeting such challenge. This situation may be generated by some social subsystems, tending to fully or partly conserve their current states. This leads to their relevant axiomatics increasing in its importance, - i.e., to the axiomatics becoming 'hyperfunctional,' which, in turn, increases the sensitivity of these subsystems to minor disturbances generated by their environment if these disturbances can be 'read' by these groups as concerning or threatening their most valuable axioms and the related practises. The result is the communicative processes within such subsystems, switched from the dissipative, diffusing HS- to the 'burning,' LS-regime. Groups dominated by information processing in this regime tend to monotonically organised, markedly linear attractors - in the form of cognitive axioms and conversion modes - capable of inducing imbalance in related social system. Therefore, the interactions of such groups with environment add in monotony and intensity - that is, aggressiveness becomes a more prominent feature of their mentality and practises. The axioms to-be-preserved act as efficient selectors in processing the information received, which may enhance suggestive mode in interpretation, thus further increasing the sensitivity of the system. Such interpreting activity amplifies any small bias that can be implied in a message from environment, and switching-on of memory structures, under the conditions, is likely to produce the same effect. All in all, this leads to specific symmetry spreading in communicative processes - within suggestion-implying messages and between such messages and the axiomatics of sociomental groups: a kind of 'metasymmetry' emerges to dominate in transferring and receiving information. Sometimes it can even cause the semantic resonance effects arising in interactions between different sociomental groups, and, thus, produce conflicts between such social subsystems. Then, social evolution approaches criticality.

Another possible route to critical regime is, again, the semantic resonance, with subsequent disturbances in social practices, but this time caused by eventual collision of distinct interpretation modes that previously worked for different social registers - e.g., for the official and the 'real-life' spheres (cf. R. D. Stacey on an organisation in the phase transition at the edge of chaos due to the legitimate and shadow systems operating against each other (1996:177). The outcome of the critical regime will depend on the nonlinearity resources in the larger society - that is, on the emergence of local, 'nuclear' solutions in the form of reshaped or drastically new axioms and conversion modes, and on their invading social subsystems rapidly enough so as to allow for the transformation in the range of possible attractors suggesting evolutionary directions for the society in question. If the social system fails to get contaminated by newly suggested cognitive axioms and conversion models rapidly enough to overcome the instability barrier, it may be destroyed and its remnants will, again, be forced to go through the nucleation of reconsidered axioms and reconstructed conversions. Therefore, it should be marked out that, within the framework of a given culture, the dominant types of conversion, incorporating certain established types of activities, may fix the related axiomatics in the minds of their agents and become, in the course of social evolution, to function as the principal constraints for the further growth and development of the culture. Another constraining factor and an important contributor to the possible emergence of the blow-up regime is a social subsystem's 'will to isolation.'

6.2. Some Common Outcomes of Communication Crisis

Outlined below is a possible 'field of evolutionary routes' (I. Prigogine's term) leading away from a social criticality regime.

6.2.1. Communicative Revolution

This is a 'violent' way to overcome dissipative tendencies in communicative crisis and to break through self-evolving trends and regularities in a social system. The agents of communicative revolution strive to impose new constraints on a social system - in the form of new axioms and conversion models. In the course of such transition forced upon the system, the social majority or minority, whose axioms and conversions do not fall in positive resonance with the privileged new axiomatics and interactions, will be isolated from their habitual external energy sources, with their conversions thus prevented from normal functioning. Within such system, the dominating mode of communicative processes and information spreading is an LS-regime ('burning'), where suggestion-implying messages prevail. This leads to enhancing the 'metasymmetry' between messages and the privileged axioms in audiences' minds. Such process obviously must strip the system of its information-rich structures, while imposing new uniformity and thus decreasing the probability for dissipative tendencies to be induced. But as mental structures and conversion practices, nonresonant with the new privileged ones, cannot be momentarily assimilated through topologically correct integration, some chaotic factors still operate at the lowest, everyday level of the related private lives, thus remaining the potential source for the future dissipation.

6.2.2. Communicative Jump

This transition is stimulated by its dire necessity, which should be widely acknowledged, and determined by its particular mechanism, which should be generally and essentially agreed upon, across the subsystems of a society. In such case, the asymptotic invariant solutions for the new social state to be attained are usually suggested at the lowest, 'nuclei' level of social life, within everyday practises of individual conversions and then start to diffuse through the larger system and thus to get it sufficiently activated to perform the jump required. The structures at the elementary level - axioms and conversion interactions - evolve from initially displaying distant correlations to finally integrating in topologically correct multilevel ensembles - new sociomental groups. In such systems, information processes are going primarily in HS-regime, which allows society to explore its potentials and capabilities and maintain the sufficient degree of nonlinearity, thus reducing the functions of, and the need for, suggestion-implying communication. Still, it is possible for a particular society to perform such jump-like transition toward the prevailing uniformity of its constituting minds, on convention or indifference on the part of overwhelming majority. In such case, the need for suggestion-implying communication may increase exponentially.

6.2.3. Communicative Stylisation

This is an attempt to jump back on some previously abandoned evolutionary route, for the sake of attaining a temporary stability. Certain ancestral communicative modes are being restored, with the underlying cognitive axioms which, though mainly stripped of their preexisting, full-fledged functions, can still serve as order factors sustaining familiar, recovered behaviour in the form of the publicly agreed upon, outward ritual. The choice of an 'axiom-behavior' precedent sample is evidently based on once-existing topologically correct organisation generated by such combination of mental and practical activities. Restorations of this kind can be 'read' as attempts at secluding from the influence of information-rich structures and thus avoiding, for a time, the impact of stochasticity by conserving mental, spatial, and time symmetry within social processes. Such situation abundantly allows for the currency of suggestion-implying information through LS-like communicative modes to prop up the artificially imposed equilibrium and reduce the system time dependence. In this case, switching on the collective memory structures enhances the social system symmetry, where coherence is attained through selection based on resonance with the privileged mental and practical patterns, serving as 'proclaimed' attractors for public activities.

6.2.4. Communicative Isolation

Such situation, politically corresponding to autarchic regime, emerges when part of a society or the whole of it secludes itself from the broader environment to satisfy a naturally evoked or imposed need for conserving the commonly adopted axiomatics and conversion modes, thus keeping them functioning as order factors. Time-independent dynamics, dominating within such society, will be sustained, in particular, by LS-regime in communication, promoted through suggestion-implying modes. Similar to communicative stylisation, communicative isolation provides for decrease in the influence of stochastic factors, especially, of information-rich structures and dissipative mode of information transferring. The difference is that in communicative isolation the axioms are supposed to be fully functional, at least, for the people in the lower part of a social hierarchy. The publicly adopted and perpetuated axiomatics works as a powerful selector, maintaining relevantly resonant, symmetric structures in mental and practical activities, while serving as strong constraints that suppress, through related social mechanisms, the nonresonant ways of thinking and acting. Thus, coherence in behaviour is reached through establishing bound, convergent relations encompassing the social system. Such communicative regime, aimed at conserving the uniform steady state once attained, favours monotonous increasing of entropy within the social system, but with living and conscious agents involved in the process, we can suppose that countertendencies will eventually emerge. Such anti-entropy tendencies can be supported by the very properties inherent to conservative dynamics - reversibility and enhanced sensitivity to any internal stochastic fluctuations or perturbations caused by environment.

6.3. Pedagogical and Didactological Systems and Needs as Order Factors in Social Context

Pedagogical and didactological systems present the structures displaying, and the factors inducing, the most conservative dynamics in societal communicative processes. Their main task is to keep cultural and, in particular, semantic tradition vigorous and functioning - that is, to sustain long-range correlations in the axiomatics adopted and the conversion modes practiced across various social subsystems and different generations, as to make communication between them possible. Ideally, in a given society, pedagogical and didactological structures function as a powerful systemic information and interpretation selector, to form such motivation and axiomatics within the minds of the persons educated that could then 'naturally' stimulate them to build the conversion modes desirable for related sociomental groups. The privileged axiomatic and conversion models serve as attractors for social practices and keep influencing and thus educating, to a greater or lesser degree, almost any agent, in his or her mental activities and practical interactions with environment throughout the agent's lifetime (cf. James Paul Gee on learning the 'right' cultural models in the course of social practices, 1999:305). The famous metaphor saying that a disciple is not a vessel to be filled, but a beacon to be ignited, seems to provide a useful insight in the general educational communicative mode which, in fact, is supposed to be most efficient when going in LS-like regime, thus necessarily favouring suggestion-implying information transfer.

6.4. Communicative Cycles

The possibility of a cyclical evolutionary route is known to be inherent in the very nature of nonlinear systems and, indeed, this type of evolution can be observed in the histories of numerous social systems (cf. I. Wallerstein on cyclical rhythm of social processes in modern world-system (2004)). This is expressed, on the practical level, in recurrence of certain preexisting conversion modes and, on the mental level, in restoration of particular preexisting axioms to their full function. Naturally, this recurrence is not reduced to mere iteration - the modes restored are necessarily adapted to variations in environmental conditions. Still, the latter play the role of selecting factors - their reproduction, in the course of a society's history, causes the agents to 'fall back' to previously found mental and practical solutions which once proved to be successful. The patterns reactivated match the external situation evidently so as to form, or to approach to, topologically correct 'agent-environment' interactive structures. The mechanism is essentially akin to imprinting (described in biology) and the 'metal memory'. The evolution of a given social system thus may tend to recur to certain privileged attractors, resonant with some structures in mental and practical activities, invariantly or periodically favoured by the society (cf. the concepts of cyclical evolution in history, elaborated e.g., by P. Sorokin (1957), and A. Schlezinger-jr. (1986)).

Conclusion

Cognitive axioms may be viewed as akin to M. Gell-Mann's schemata - which contain some information compressed to 'predict the environment' and work as 'kinds of cultural DNA' (see Lewin 1992:15). Ralph D. Stacey, elaborating on the nature of such schemata, writes that they are extracted from the models of the world, built on environmental feedback on the consequences of behaviour (1996:21). In Adrian Baddeley's view, such schemata may work as 'behavioural scripts, evaluative rules, or mental models' and regulate the search for, and interpretation of, the information coming and the actions consequently undertaken (1990, in Stacey 1996:30, cf. M. Mitchell Waldrop on 'internal models of the world' as 'the building blocks of behavior,' 1993:146). These rules form the part of shared culture and may be embodied in social institutions (Stacey 1996:32).

But it is important to note that cognitive axioms essentially are not the sets of well-structured thoughts but rather 'self-evident,' often unconscious or half-conscious mental units guiding actions. The significance of the mental structures of this kind was emphasised by the researcher in organisations as dynamical systems, Gareth Morgan: 'The hidden and sometimes unquestioned assumptions that are built in the design of information systems can be of crucial importance in structuring day-to-day activity' (1997:180). Such axioms quite often operate in 'implicit models' of the world, without humans being aware of these operations (cf. Waldrop 1993:178-179). Cognitive axioms can be viewed as kind of low-level rules which can be transferred as generalised genotype (C. Langton's term in Waldrop 1993:281), primarily, in the course of education and activated as generalised phenotype (C. Langton's term in Waldrop 1993:281) in a matching environment. Cognitive axioms may provide for constraints and self-organisation in human minds and social systems and, when widely shared, act as important contributors to societal stability and, thus, predictability. It should be noted, though, that the quality of axioms-based social stability may radically differ, as differ the qualities of the axioms themselves and the minds of their agents. Individually adopted axioms, to the contrary, provide for chaotic behaviour and unpredictability on the social scale, like in a case termed 'social atomization.'

Cognitive axioms also make it possible to trace sense links in complex human behaviour, even if the causal links are lost to an observer of behavioural complexity (cf. Stacey 1996:67-68). Some cognitive axioms may be at the core of social adaptation process (cf. Stacey 1996:90), thus forming the body of ontogenetic, individual a priori knowledge which is shaped and accumulated in the course of philogenetic, species evolution (cf. 'dominant schemas' - e.g., in Stacey 1996:101). Still, cognitive axioms are not an absolutely static material. Sometimes, they can be changed, rearranged, substituted or even dropped in the course of an individual or sociomental group evolution (cf. M. Mitchell Waldrop on 'internal models of the world' as 'implicit and explicit assumptions' about environment, 1993:146). It is important, then, that cognitive axioms should rather neatly combine the tendency to evolve with the tendency to conserve as to make it possible for a living system to move on without desintegrating too soon. Christopher Langton pointed at the possibility that, at the edge of chaos, 'information processing can become an important part of the dynamics of the system' (see Lewin 1992:51). With living systems, it seems to be a crucial factor for their existing and properly functioning in environment, which helps them to 'tune their interactions' and thus to 'hone the ability to evolve' (Lewin 1992:59) and adapt.

An important point about axioms-based communication is that its mechanism evidently integrates the elements of LS-regime, contrary to the normal view regarding the information transferring as essentially an HS-regime process.

Happily formulated, explicitly adopted and widely shared axiom can promote a phase transition in a society. That is what Brian Arthur writes about: 'It turns out that an awful lot of policy-making has to do with finding the appropriate metaphor. Conversely, bad policy-making almost always involves finding inappropriate metaphors' (in Waldrop 1993:334). It should be noted, though, that cognitive axioms do not necessarily always take on the form of metaphors. At least, more often than not, they are not regarded as metaphors by people who adopt them as guidance in their activities.

Providing a sufficient amount of field data, the concept presented could be used in modelling a way or a style of life as complex dynamical system.

References

Allport, G. (1954) *The nature of prejudice*. Cambridge: Addison-Wesley.

Aronson, E. (1995) *The social animal*. (7th ed.) New York, NY: W. H. Freeman and Company.

Basar, E., Flohr, H., & Haken, H. (Eds.) (1983) *Synergetics of brain*. Berlin: Springer.

Berger, J. A., & Heath, C. (2005) How the prevalence of environment cues influences the success of ideas. *Cognitive Science*, 29 (2):195-221.

Bettinghaus, E. P. (1980) *Persuasive communication*. (3rd ed.) New York, NY: Holt, Rinehart & Winston.

Cialdini, R. B. (2001) *Influence: Science and practice*. (4th ed.) Boston, MA: Allyn & Bacon.

Dreymanis, A. P. (1987) *Neurosynergetics and the process of creative thinking* [Нейросинергетика и процесс творческого мышления]. In *Scientific technical creativity: Problems of eurilogy* (abstracts of reports delivered at the republican conference at the Institute of Philosophy and Law) [Научно-техническое творчество: Проблемы эврилогии (тезисы доклада республиканской конференции в Институте философии и права]. (pp. 152-154) Riga: Zinatne.

Dridze, T. M. (2000) *Two new paradigms for social epistemology and social practice* [Две новые парадигмы для социального познания и социальной практики]. In T. M. Dridze (Ed.) *Social communication and governance in ecoanthropocentric and semiosociopsychological paradigms* [Социальная коммуникация и социальное управление в экоантропоцентрической и семиосоцио-психологической парадигмах]: in 2 vols. Vol. 1. (pp. 3-34) Moscow: The Institute of Sociology of the Russian Academy of Sciences.

Dunn, W. N. (1994) *Public policy analysis, an introduction.* (2nd ed.) Englewood Cliffs, CA: Prentice Hall.

Eysenck, H. J. (1982) *Personality, genetics, and behavior: selected papers*. New York: Praeger.

Farmer, J. D. (1982) Dimension, fractal measures, and chaotic dynamics. In H. Haken (Ed.) *Evolution of order and chaos in physics, chemistry, and biology: proceedings of the International Symposium on Synergetics at Schloss Elmau*, Bavaria, April 26 - May 1, 1982. Berlin, New York: Springer.

Filin, V. A. (1998) *Visual environment as a social factor* [Визуальная среда как социальный фактор]. In T. M. Dridze (Ed.) *City planning: from social diagnostics to effective dialogue of the parties involved* [Градоустройство: от социальной диагностики к конструктивному диалогу заинтересованных сторон]: in 2 vols. Vol. 1 (pp. 64-79) Moscow: The Institute of Sociology, Russian Academy of Sciences, Center for Governance, Communication, and Socioplanning Technologies RAS.

Final Report of the National Commission on Terrorist Attacks upon the United States, Official Government Edition. (2004) Section 11. Foresight and Hindsight: 11.1. Imagination (p. 1 of 22 p.). Available at: http://www.gpo.access.gov/911/index.html.

Fish, S. (1994 (1980)) Interpreting the Variorum. In R. C. Davis, & R. Schleifer (Eds.) *Contemporary literary criticism: Literary and cultural studies*. (3rd ed., pp. 175-190) New York, London: Longman.

Garfinkel, H. (1964) Studies of routine grounds of everyday activities. *Social Problems* 11 (3):220-250.

Gee, J. P. (1999) Mind and society: A response to Derek Edwards' 'Emotion Discourse.' *Culture and Psychology, Discourse Analysis: Special Issue* 5 (3):305-312.

Haken, H. (1984) Some introductory remarks on synergetics. In E. Frehland (Ed.) *Synergetics - from microscopic to macroscopic order*. Berlin: Springer.

Holsti, O. R. (1977) *The 'operational code' as an approach to analysis of belief systems.* Durham: Duke University Press.

Homans, G. K. (1961) *Social behavior: its elementary forms.* R. K. Merton (General ed.) New York: Harcourt, Brace & World.

Huxley, J. (1961) *La protection de la grande faune et des habitats naturels en Afrique centrale et orientale:*[*The protection of large fauna and natural habitats in Central and Eastern Africa*] Rapport sur une mission accomplie pour l'UNESCO (juillet - septembre 1960). Paris: UNESCO.

Jepperson, R. L., Wendt, A., & Katzenstein, P. J. (1996) Norms, identity, and culture in national security. In P J. Katzenstein (Ed.) *The culture of national security: norms and identity in world politics.* (pp. 33-75) J. G. Ruggie (General ed.) *New directions in world politics.* New York: Columbia University Press.

Kadomtsev, B. B. (1999) Dynamics and information [Динамика и информация]. (2nd ed.) Moscow: *Journal 'Uspekhi fizicheskikh nauk.'*

Kelly, G. A. (1955) *The psychology of personal constructs:* in 2 vols. New York: Norton.

Kennamer, J. D. (1989) Deceptive advertising and the power of suggestion. In T. J. Smith III (Ed.) *Propaganda, a pluralistic perspective*. (pp. 139-149) New York, etc.: Praeger.

Knyazeva, H. N., & Kurdyumov, S. P. (2002) *Foundations of synergetics. Criticality regimes, autoorganisation, tempoworlds* [Основания синергетики. Режимы с обострением, самоорганизация, темпомиры]. Sanct-Peterburg: Aleteya.

Lewin, R. (1992) *Complexity. Life at the edge of chaos*. New York: Collier Brooks, Macmillan Publ. Co.

Lioutikova, E. V. (2006) Axioms of cognition affecting human-environmental interactions as traced in historiographical texts. *The Social Science Journal*, 43 (1):35-46.

Lumsden, Ch., & Wilson, E. O. (1981) *Genes, mind, and culture, the coevolutionary process*. Cambridge: Harvard University Press.

Morgan, G. (1997) *Images of organization*. Thousand Oaks: Sage.

Moscovici, S. (1985) *The Age of the Crowd: A Historical Treatise on Mass Psychology*. Transl. by J. C. Whitehouse. Cambridge, New York: Cambridge University Press, Paris: Editions de la Maison des Sciences de l'Homme.

Nazaretyan, A. P. (1996) *Agression, morals, and crises in development of the world culture* (The synergetics of historic process): *The lecture course* [Агрессия, мораль и кризисы в развитии мировой культуры (Синергетика исторического процесса). Курс лекций]. (2nd ed., rev. and amend.) Moscow: Naslediye.

Nechayev, V. D. (2002) *Cognitive revolutions and institutional changes* [Когнитивные революции и институциональные изменения]. Polis (5):6-19.

Nolan, M. A., Haslam, S. A., Spears, R., & Oakes, P. J. (1999) An examination of resource-based and fit-based theories of stereotyping under cognitive load and fit. *European Journal of Social Psychology*, 29 (5/6): 641-663.

Nurkova, V. V. (2000) *Present perfect: Psychology of personal autobiographical memory* [Свершенное продолжается: Психология автобиографической памяти личности]. Moscow: The University of Russian Academy of Education.

O'Donnell, V., & Jowett, G. S. (1989) Propaganda as the form of communication. In T. J. Smith III (Ed.) *Propaganda, a pluralistic perspective*. (pp. 49-63) New York, etc.: Praeger.

Petty, R. E., & Cacioppo, J. T. (1981) *Attitudes and persuasion: Classic and contemporary approaches*. Dubuque: Wm. C. Brown.

Reymers, N. F. (1994) Ecology (theories, laws, rules, principles, and hypotheses) [Экология (теории, законы, правила, принципы и гипотезы)]. Moscow: *Journal 'Rossiya molodaya.'*

Ricoeur, P. (1974) *The conflict of interpretations*. Ed. by D. Ihde. Evanston: Northwestern University Press.

Rokeach, M. (1972) *Beliefs, attitudes, and values, a theory of organization and change*. San Francisco, etc.: Jossey-Bass Inc.

Rottenstreich, Y., & Tversky, A. (1997) Unpacking, repacking, and anchoring: Advances in support theory. *Psychological Review*, 104 (2):406-415.

Salmon, N. (1988) How to measure the standard metre. *Proceedings of the Aristotelian Society* (New Series), vol. 88, pp. 193-217.

Schlezinger, A. M., Jr. (1986) *The cycles of American history*. Boston: Houghton Mifflin.

Sherif, C., Sherif, M., & Nebergall, R. (1965) *Attitude and attitude change*: *The social judgment-involvement approach*. Philadelphia: W. B. Saunders.

Simon, H. A. (1967) The logic of heuristic decision making. In N. Rescher (Ed.). *The logic of decision and action* (pp. 1-20). Pittsburgh: University of Pittsburgh Press.

Sorokin, P. (1957) *Social and cultural dynamics: a study of change in major systems of art, truth, ethics, law, and social relationships.* (Rev. and abr. by the author) Boston: Extending Horizons Books.

Stacey, R. D. (1996) *Complexity and creativity in organizations*. San Francisco: Beret-Koehler Publ.

Tajfel, H. (1981) *Human groups and social categories*. Cambridge: Cambridge Univ. Press.

Turkulets, A. V. (2002) Subjects of social cognition [Субъекты социального познания]. *Nauchnaya mysl Kavkaza*, (2): 49-57.

Tversky, A., & Kahneman, D. (1973) Availability: A heuristic for judging frequency and probability. *Cognitive Psychology*, 5 (2):207-232.

Tversky, A., & Koehler, D. J. (1994) Support theory: A nonextensional representation of subjective probability. *Psychological Review*, 101 (4):547-567.

Vergiles, N. Yu., & Andreyeva, Ye. A. (1998) *Once again on the mechanisms of visual perception* [Ещё раз о механизмах работы зрительного восприятия]. In A. V. Brushlinskyi et al. (Eds.) *Mental representation: dynamics and structure* [Ментальная репрезентация: динамика и структура]. (pp. 277-290) Moscow: The Institute of Psychology, Russian Academy of Sciences.

Waldrop, M. M. (1993) Complexity. The emerging science at the edge of order and chaos. *A Touchstone Book.* New York, London, etc.: Simon & Schuster.

Wallerstein, I. (2004) *World-system analysis: an introduction*. Durham: Duke University Press.

Winograd, T. (1977) A framework for understanding discourse. In M. A. Just, & P. E. Carpenter (Eds.) *Cognitive processes in comprehension.* (pp. 63-68) Hillsdale: Lawrence Erlbaum.

Zimbardo, P. G., & Leippe, M. R. (1991) *The psychology of attitude change and social influence.* Boston, etc: McGraw Hill.

Chapter 5

Mind Force Theory: Hyper-Network Dynamics in Neuroscience*

Franco Orsucci†
Department of Neurology and Behavioral Sciences, University of Siena,
Department of Psychology, University College London, UK

Abstract

A definition of Mind Force would be as the dynamical hyperstructure formed by networks of synchronized oscillators coupled in fields spanning trough heterogeneous domains. Mind Force theory is based on the integration of 4 main pillar-theories: Complexity theory; Synchronization theory; Network theory; Field theory. Mind Force is the result of the causal power of collective phenomena and patterns. Precursors and conditions for Mind Force theory are examined and a possible pathway for modeling is proposed.

Keywords: synchronization, neuroscience, language, cognition, network, mind, force

1. Introduction: Interacting Oscillators

In an interesting study Ernest Lawrence Rossi (1996) tried to draw the whole picture of the psychobiology of mind-body communication as "the complex,

---

* This article was originally published in *Chaos and Complexity Letters*, volume 4 number 3 (2010).

† Corresponding Author's Email: f.orsucci@ucl.ac.uk.

In: Neuroscience and Technology Transform the Educational Ecosystem
Editors: Franco F. Orsucci and Nicoletta Sala
ISBN: 979-8-88697-157-6

self-organizing field of information transduction." Unfortunately, at the time, he missed most of the contemporary knowledge on synchronization, network theory and field theory, just focusing on information streams and transduction. Anyway, his attempt is interesting, especially for the figure he include which might give us some hint about the scales, clusters and processes we are going to describe as the operations of Mind Force.

It is quite evident that the resulting hypernetwork is formed by different kind of oscillators: relaxation and non-relaxation; chaotic and non-chaotic; with similar and with quite different frequencies etc. David Somers and Nancy Kopell (1995) studied waves and synchrony in networks of oscillators of relaxation and non-relaxation type. They showed how chains of phase oscillators that phase-lock produce travelling waves.

The waves were shown to be a consequence of boundary effects: the oscillators at the ends receive different input than those in the middle, and compensate for the difference by setting up phase differences. They also observed fractured waves and fractured synchrony in networks of relaxation oscillators.

Horacio Zanette has been focusing in this same area of research and in a paper with Alexander Mikhailov they studied condensation in globally coupled populations of chaotic dynamical systems (Zanette and Mikhailov, 1998 a and b). They found that synchronization begins at low coupling intensities with the appearance of small coherent groups of oscillators on the background of the rest of the population performing asynchronous oscillations. The elements belonging to such groups constitute a dynamical condensate. As the coupling strength is increased, the number of particles in the condensate grows and eventually the whole population becomes divided into several coherent clusters. Within each cluster, the elements follow the same chaotic dynamical trajectory. Under further increase of the global coupling, the number of coherent clusters gets reduced until full mutual synchronization is achieved. To quantitatively characterize the condensation, they used two order parameters. The first of them is given by the ratio r of the number of pairs with zero distances to the total number of pairs. In the absence of a condensate, r = 0. On the other hand, r = 1 when complete mutual synchronization of the whole population takes place. The second parameter s represents the fraction of the population belonging to coherent clusters. It is given by the relative number of elements that have at least one other element with the same state in the considered population. Therefore, s can be viewed as characterizing the size of the condensate.

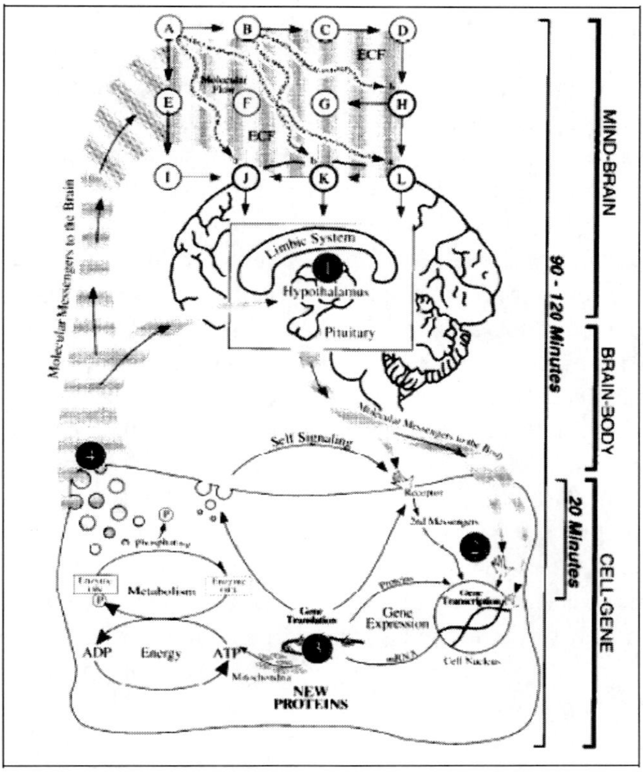

Figure 1. Heterogeneous couplings in hyperstructure (Rossi, 1996).

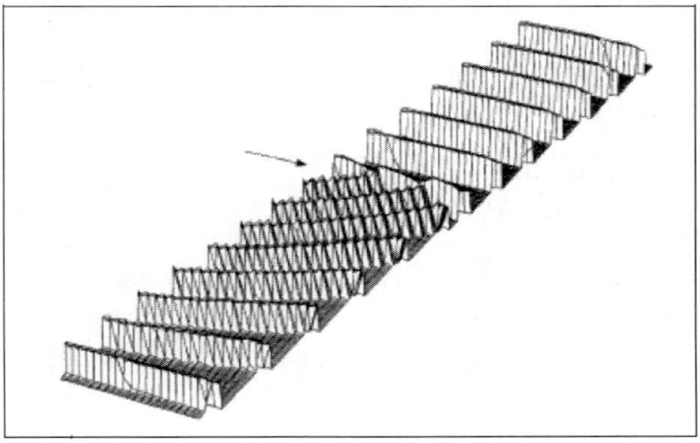

Figure 2. Start of synchrony and travelling waves in relaxation oscillators (Somers and Kopell, 1995).

These forms of synchronization are essential to the functioning of some artificial systems, and have been observed in certain insect populations. On the other hand, they are expected to play a less relevant role in most biological systems, where the complexity of collective functions requires a delicate balance between coherence and diversity. Consider, for instance, the brain, where highly coherent activity patterns are only realized under pathological states, such as during epileptic seizures. Many biological systems consisting of interacting agents, ranging from bio-molecular complexes to social populations, are normally found in configurations where the ensemble is segregated into groups with specific functions (Zanette and Mikhailov 2004).

While the evolution of individual elements is highly correlated inside each group, the collective dynamics of different groups is much more independent. Usually, clustering is a dynamical process, where groups may preserve their identity in spite of the fact that single elements are continuously migrating between them. The individual motion towards or away from clusters may also be controlled by the internal state of each element, which favors or inhibits grouping with other elements. This is observed in natural phenomena ranging from complex chemical reactions, where biomolecules react with each other only when they have reached appropriate internal configurations, to social systems, where the appearance of organizational structures requires compatibility between the individual changing states of the involved agents. The behavior of each single oscillator is usually described in terms of differential equations which can be linear or non linear (the latter usually for biological oscillators). Nonlinear dynamics is the study of the complex ways a system evolves over time. The collective behavior of enormous systems of units has been usually described by statistical mechanics. Network theory is a way to connect these complimentary branches of physics. The analytical techniques of statistical physics can be brought to bear the puzzle of how brain cells and other living things mange to synchronize each other (Strogatz 2003: 55; Albert and Barabasi 2002). Like light in quantum theory, oscillators can be considered as sine waves or as particles. Networks of oscillators could be modeled as spin glasses, or spin foam. We may even recognize how ensembles of oscillators and networks might present peculiar quantum phenomena like the Bose-Einstein condensate, a spontaneous collapse into the same quantum state, the state of lower possible energy (Strogatz 2003: 134). In this state all the waves are locked in step, they are phase coherent.

2. Precursors

Remarkably little has been written about consciousness in the theory of biological evolution. Richards (1987) captures the core of the problem in his summing up of an argument originally formulated by William James (1996).

"Consciousness is a manifest trait of higher organisms, most perspicuously of man; like all such traits it must have evolved; yet it could have evolved only if it were naturally selected; but if naturally selected it must have a use; and if it have a use, then it cannot be causally inert. Mind, therefore must be more than an excretion of brain; it must be, at least in some respect an independently effective process that is able to control some central nervous activity" (Richards, 1987: 431). We might add that mind must have a power control over the effectiveness of man on reality.

The idea that an immaterial entity can influence a material entity (reality and the body) is not compatible with an old notion of causality according to which every change in the natural world is produced by contact of spatially extended bodies. This argument was raised by many of Descartes contemporaries. Their primitive antiquated conception of matter as something spatially extended and the related connected notion of causality (as restricted to action by contact) was outpaced by subsequent developments in physics. This conception has not entirely lost its influence in scientific debate and common views. For example P. S. Churchland argues against the existence of "soul stuff" that is not "spatially extended" (1986: 318). Dennett discusses what he calls the *standard objection* which was all too familiar to Descartes (Descartes, 1988; Dennett, 1991) reformulating it in modern terms. In his illustration of this modern criticism, we find the paradox of *Casper the Friendly Ghost* who is both gliding through walls and grabbing falling towels. These contradictory events seem more of a problem for the adherents of mechanistic notions than to those who are familiar with modern physics.

The *analogy* between mind and forces is not an entirely new concept. In philosophy, Hobbes and Leibniz identified a component of mind which they called *conatus,* with a physical force.

3. Fields

In different ways, some of the key founders of modern psychology, such as Sigmund Freud, William James and Carl Jung, were presenting issues in favor of Mind Force (MF). The history of this construct was progressing during the following years.

During the late 40s, a social psychologist, Kurt Lewin (1890-1947) born in Germany, immigrated to the USA because of World War II. He established also the Research Center for Group Dynamics at Massachusetts Institute of Technology. Lewin stated that: 'One should view the present situation—the *status quo*—as being maintained by certain conditions or forces' (Lewin, 1943a: 172). Lewin, who was well known for using concepts like *life space* and *field theory*, proposed to view the social environment as a dynamic field affecting human consciousness. In turn, the person's psychological state influences the social field or milieu.

Lewin sought to describe group life, and to investigate conditions and forces, which bring about change or resist change in groups. In his field theory, a *field* is defined as 'the totality of coexisting facts which are conceived of as mutually interdependent' (Lewin 1951: 240). Lewin believed that in order for change to take place, the total situation has to be taken into account. If only part of the situation is considered, a misrepresentation of the picture is likely to develop. The whole psychological field, or *lifespace*, within which people acted, had to be viewed, in order to understand human behavior. Within this framework, individuals and groups could be seen in topological terms (using map-like representations). Individuals participate in a series of life spaces, (such as the family, work, school and church) and these spaces were constructed under the influence of various force vectors (Lewin 1952). His active approach could be summarized in his motto: "Learning is more effective when it is an active rather than a passive process: if you want to truly understand something, try to change it" (Lewin, 1952).

Harry S. Sullivan (1892 – 1949), like Lewin, was concerned about using theoretical constructs featuring falsifiable reference in interpersonal behavior. While Sullivan may not have read Lewin, Wertheimer, Kohler, or Koffka, he almost certainly would have had welcomed their general approach, since he was proposing a psychological field theory similar to their psycho-physical field theory. He may have seriously intended only a loose heuristic function in casting interpersonal relations as occurring in a "field." Nevertheless, he was intrigued by this notion. It seemed to him that the field provided an accurate and useful description of effects. Though he didn't write much about fields and mind force, during his brief lifespan, he left a wonderful sketch presented during one of his last lectures (LaForge, 2004).

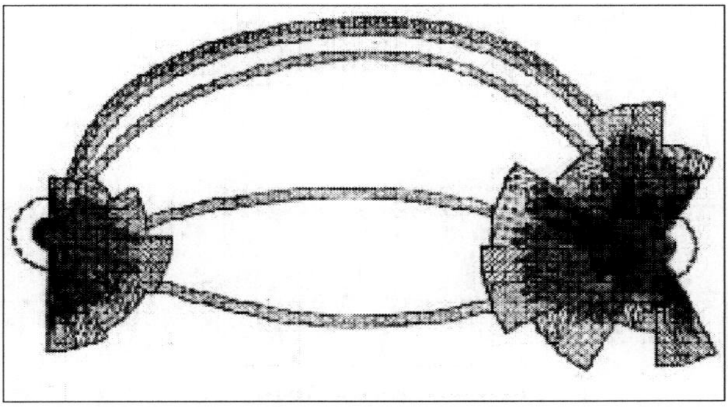

Figure 3. H. S. Sullivan sketch on mind force fields in a couple (LaForge, 2004).

4. Force

More recently, the philosopher Karl Popper has emphasized the similarities between mind and forces: "Minds are located, unextended, incorporeal, capable of acting on bodies, dependent on body and capable of being influenced by bodies. (…) Now, I say, things of this kind *do* exist, and we all know it. So, what are these things? These things are forces" (Popper, 1993: 168).

Popper seems to go further than a mere analogy, and he proposes, as a hypothesis "that the complicated electro-magnetic wave fields which, as we know, are part of the physiology of our brains, represent the unconscious part of our minds, and that the conscious mind – our conscious mental intensities, our conscious experiences – are capable of interacting with this unconscious physical force fields, especially when problems *need* to be solved. That *need* is what we call *attention*" (Popper, 1993: 179).

Here Popper is considering unconscious as synonymous with the physical force fields. In the figure in the following page, you might notice that there is an area of mind/brain overlap. This area represents a form of biophysical unconscious. Popper points out that conscious mind may "sink into physiology" and become unconscious: "a mergent process, a process where (unconscious) mind and brain are no longer distinguishable" (Popper 1993: 171).

In explaining part of his conception of unconscious, Popper utilized the example of learning a complex psychomotor skill (playing the piano, grasping a mug, and a lot of other activities). In the first stages of the learning process we are conscious and our attention is focused on each single step in the new skills to learn. This stage, sooner or later, disappears and we no longer think about each single step. The new acquired skills are now embodied and, we might say, merged in our being. This process is part of the constitution of *procedural memory*.

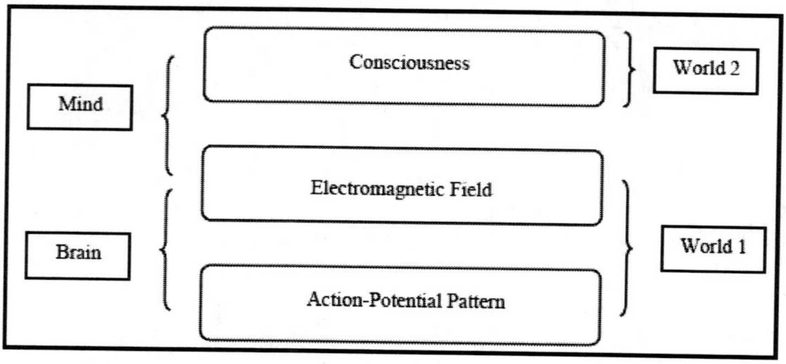

Figure 4. Karl Popper's scheme.

There is no need to postulate a mind force in order to explain procedural memory, so Popper's example might be misleading. His proposal of founding mind force on electromagnetic interactions is also improbable for physical reasons. Anyway, some of Popper remarks and his endorsement of the necessity of MF theory are certainly important.

5. Conscious Mental Fields

Benjamin Libet, in the same years, had also proposed the hypothetical existence of a *Conscious Mental Field* (CMF) (Libet 1993, 1994). The CMF would emerge as a function of neural activities in the brain and it would have the attribute of a conscious subjective experience. Libet also suggested that it could act back on certain neural activities and would therefore affect behavior, as in a willed action. It would account for the unity of a subjective experience, even though the latter emerges from the myriad of activities of billions of nerve cells and their synaptic and non-synaptic interplays.

In Libet's opinion "The CMF, like the subjective experiences constituted in it, would be accessible only to the individual having the experiences it could not be directly observed by any external physical device except indirectly, by any effects it introduces on behavioral outcomes (just as conscious will is evidenced)" (Libet, 1996: 223).

In a paper entitled "Mind as a force field: a new interactionistic hypothesis," B. Lindahl and P. Arhem (1994) proposed a critical review of some modern approaches to Mind Force. Libet in his response to their remarks (1996) wrote that he liked "Popper's idea of viewing the mind as a kind of force field." Such a CMF force would have been different from all known physical forces, though Popper's hypothesis does not appear to spell out any attributes of that conscious physical force field except in its ability to interact with another entity. The electromagnetic field representing the unconscious mental functions is "doubtful based on evidence available." Consciousness, following Libet's experiments, can simply be a function of the duration of cerebral activations to achieve awareness. Libet was stressing that, "Evidence suggests that conscious functions involve some special neural activities that are simply added to those involved in conscious functions" (1996: 224). Libet is posing two important questions: first, how does the CMF arise out of mental activities; and second, exactly how the CMF does act on the physical brain.

Nevertheless, it seems that Libet was forgetting the dynamical nature of CMF and the self-organizing nature of its power. He does revisit the issue, reminding, "whether electromagnetic fields are representative of unconscious mental functions could be tested in principle by experimentally distorting and/or disrupting or modifying such fields in the putative relation to unconscious functions." Sperry (1947) had already tried such experiment by cutting the monkey cortex in slices. However, Sperry's vertical cuts in the cortex may not have affected larger field currents as electrical pathways over and below the cuts were still present as a potential role for over-arching electric fields therefore remains possible.

6. The Aconscious

Lindahl and Arhem (1996) noted that "in the mental force field hypothesis only the unconscious part of mind is explicitly interpreted in field terms." They correctly point out that Libet (1996) mistakenly assumed that the Popper force field hypothesis applied to the conscious mind. Popper left open the question of the nature of conscious mind However; he did except to say that the mind in its general form emerges from the body, somehow, but is not reducible to it. What Libet misunderstood, and it might be not clear enough in Lindahl and Arhem response, is that the unconscious in question should be properly named *aconscious.* Its contents and processes are not repressed, and possibly recalled to consciousness, but rather embedded in the human psychomotor structure via psycho-physiological storage.

Libet, more recently (2006), has summarized his view on Mind Force. He starts recognizing that, if there is a generally held assumption that mind and brain can interact, this indicates that "two phenomenological entities exist." After this "back to Descartes" statement, he continues with the questionable assumption that mind, in his view, is just a subjective experience, accessible only by individual introspection.

This point of view, discards all the psychological and linguistic research studying psychomotor, perceptual and linguistic manifestations or derivatives of mind functioning. His point recalls the "private language" paradox proposed by Ludwig Wittgenstein (1967). The conclusion raised by this paradox is that every form of language and thinking (even the so-called inner dialogue) relies on our shared forms of communication. Language (also in the form of culture) is pre-existing to the subject, though its communicative or private usage for thinking can be personalized. If the idea of a private language is incoherent, then it would follow that all language is essentially public: that language is at its core a social phenomenon. For instance, if one cannot have a private language, it might not make any sense to talk of private sensations such as *qualia*; nor might it make sense to talk of a word as referring to a concept, if a concept is understood to be a private mental representation.

Libet recalls the interest that Sir John Eccles derived from Sir Charles Sherrington for the interactions between brain and mind. When the physicist, Henry Margenau, provided a view of the mind as a field that could interact with the brain even with no energy expenditure (Margenau, 1984), this supported Eccles' bias on the nature of mind–brain interaction.

Libet notes, "It is especially noteworthy that Eccles' models of mind–brain interaction were presented without any experimental evidence or experimental designs for testing. That was due at least partly to the untestability of the models. Curiously, an absence of experimental testability did not bother Eccles. When asked if his view that a field of ''psychons'' (his units of mental function; see Wiesendanger, 2006) could mediate the unity of subjective experience (Eccles, 1990) was untestable, Eccles replied that he knew of no way to test that hypothesis (personal communication). Nevertheless, he argued that the hypothesis had explanatory power, and, as such, he believed it had some usefulness and even validity. Eccles produced a stimulus further contribution to work in the direction of an MF definition, but his models remained untested, and, apparently, he was not bothered about it.

Libet raises the testability issue also about the approach proposed by Hiromi Umezawa and his followers: as they proposed a mental field model, which they termed a *Quantum Field Theory* (claimed by this group of authors as different from *Quantum Mechanics*) (Ricciardi and Umezawa, 1967; Umezawa and Vitiello, 1986; Vitiello, 1995; 2001; 2002). In Libet's opinion, "Their model is mostly mathematical, however, and it is not clear how it can be tested" (Libet, 1993; Libet, Freeman and Sutherland, 1999). Libet is raising a similar objection against the quantum mechanics approach as in the interpretation of quantum theory by Nils Bohr (1885–1962) mind and matter are two aspects of one undivided process. David Böhm (1917–1992) adopted this idea (see Böhm and Factor, 1985). However, this does not solve the problem of how the neuronal activity aspect relates to the subjective, non-physical aspect of mind. If subjective experience is a non-physical phenomenon, what is it? The merit of the Bohr-Böhm approach is in recognizing that there is a physical process behind and beyond mind and brain.

Libet claims that his CMF theory is potentially testable as he described a design for conducting such tests. The proposed experimental test is simple in principle but difficult to carry out, a small slab of sensory cortex, which keeps the tiny cortex island alive by preserving the blood vessels providing blood flow from the arterial branches that dip vertically into the cortex. "The prediction is that electrical stimulation of the sensory slab will produce a subjective response reportable by the subject. That is, activity in the isolated slab can contribute by producing its own portion of the CMF." (Libet, 2006: 324). He states, and we agree with him, that his CMF is an emergent and localizable system property. Less clear is why this experiment, which doesn't seem technically so difficult, has not been performed yet by other scientists or Libet himself.

Libet is also referring to the functioning of the CMF as the delay in sensory awareness of 0.5 s after the initial response of the cortex as well as the other very interesting phenomenon related to readiness for action, which is preceding actual actions by about 300 ms. So, both perceptual and motor activities have significant delays with consciousness. *These empirical findings support the autonomy of aconscious Mind Force processes from consciousness processes.* This landmark, (though still partially controversial) findings by Libet, could entirely re-design the role of conscious and unconscious processes. The term unconscious here can be mistakenly confused with the traditional (repressed) unconscious, but in this case, we are dealing with events without any conscious representation. Indeed, most mental events are unconscious, or we might better say, *aconscious* (Orsucci, 2002b;

Orsucci, 2002a). Libet concludes his review mentioning in vivo and brain imaging research supporting his findings. “If an experimental test of the CMF was to be carried out, like that described above, it might confirm or contradict the kind of alternatives possible for a mind–brain interaction” (Libet, 2006: 326).

7. Energy

Walter J Freeman, after his explorations on mass action in the nervous system, chaos dynamics in perception and social dynamics, has more recently proposed a Mind Force approach (Freeman, 2007). He first defines the framework of this approach: “Consciousness fully supervenes when the 1.5 kgm mass of protoplasm in the head directs the body into material and social environments and engages in reciprocity. While consciousness is not susceptible to direct measurement, a limited form exercised in animals and pre-lingual children can be measured indirectly with biological assays of arousal, intention and attention.” It is a remarkably non-deterministic and interactionistic approach.

After a general description of the multiple levels of interactions involved, from the molecular to the social levels, including their intermingling, he states: “Every reflex and intentional act and thought is based on the exchanges of matter and energy through neural activity at every scale.” (Freeman, 2007: 1022). There is a need for a universal language to comprehend all the incredible mesh of interactions involved and the mathematical tools needed might be already at hand,.

There is no definition of what consciousness is and, no physiological or cognitive index of consciousness, as many discussions on consciousness still tend to confuse it with self-consciousness. So, Freeman states that he wants to consider the perceptual and behavioral derivates of consciousness that we might find even in infants and animals, “I leave the hard problem (Chalmers, 1995) to philosophers.”

He stresses that the stream of consciousness is cinematographic, as we have seen in chapter 2 rather than continuous. Consciousness role in human behavior is judgmental rather than enactive, so that its prime role is not to make decisions but to delay and defer action and thereby minimize premature commitment of limited resources. Just as we use to say in the adage, “stop and think before acting.” Following this path, Freeman comes to a clear statement: “consciousness is not merely ‘like’ a force; it is a field of force that can be understood in the same ways that we understand all other fields of force within which we, through our bodies, are immersed, and which we, through our bodies, comprehend in accordance with the known laws of physics." (Freeman, 2007: 1022).

The models that Freeman has implemented are schematized in two ways: one is the so called Katchalsky model (or K-sets) (Freeman, 1975; Kozma and Freeman, 2003); the other one is the quantum field model he more recently developed in collaboration with Giuseppe Vitiello (2006).

In Freeman's description Mind Force might be found in the action–perception cycle as described by Piaget (1930) and Merleau-Ponty (1942). The cycle begins with a macroscopic state in the brain that embodies a goal. It emerges in the brain from a predictive state implicitly containing nested mesoscopic activity patterns, constructed in corticostriatal and corticocerebellar modules (Houk, 2005). The predictive expectations embedded in sensory cortices are described as landscapes of chaotic attractors within the brain state space. The dynamic memory embodied in nerve cell assemblies is manifested in spatial pattern of amplitude modulation, mostly in the gamma band range.

An interesting property of the system is that these dynamical landscapes lack invariance, as they change whether the same stimulus is reinforced or not, or the context is different or the sequence of stimuli is different.

"The attractor governs the neural interactions that generate an oscillatory field of neural activity called a wave packet" (Freeman, 1975). Fields are not fixed representations of the stimuli, and stimuli are not grounded in any fixed way. Each action-perception frame is separated from the others by phase transitions. Freeman cites Wolfgang Köhler who was (1940: 55) quite explicit about this: "Our present knowledge of human perception leaves no doubt as to the general form of any theory which is to do justice to such knowledge: *a theory of perception must be a field theory*.

By this we mean that the neural functions and processes with which the perceptual facts are associated in each case are located in a continuous medium." Regrettably, Köhler identified his perceptual field with the epiphenomenal electric field of the EEG, of which the Coulomb forces are much too weak to synchronize the observed oscillations in wave packets. Sperry (1980) and Pribram (1971) easily disproved this subsidiary hypothesis, with the unfortunate outcome that mainstream neuroscientists largely abandoned field hypotheses.

8. Four Pillars

Complexity theory has provided the empirical and mathematical tools to prove that the brain patterns correlated to the cine-like frames in the action-perception cycle are like bubbles in a pan of boiling water at the critical temperature. They can be seen also as the avalanches on a sand pile, as in the model of *self-organized criticality* proposed by Per Bak (Bak et al., 1978; Bak, 1990; Bak, 1996).

From this neurodynamical point of view, the personal identity is "embodied in the entirety of the brain-body dynamics" this is the reason why we have been speaking about a comprehensive *biophysical identity*. We find this definition more grounded and explicit, but in the same line of the approach suggested, with different nuances, as *embodiment* (Varela, Thompson, and Rosch, 1991), *proto-self* (Damasio, 1999), *synaptic self* (LeDoux, 2002). Following the history of the Mind Force construct we might realize how it come comes gradually to take the shape of a new theory, approaching the stage in which it can be formalized. We can summarize some of the necessary prerequisites of this theory.

In order to recognize the existence and operability of MF and its related phenomena, we need to accept and stabilize a definitive transcending of the notorious Cartesian dichotomy. The current discussion on Descartes' error is often missing two important points: the heuristic value that his position has had for centuries in the advancement of science; and a full recognition of all the implications that discarding his approach will have on our new scientific approaches. MF is beyond *Res Cogitans* and *Res Extensa* in dynamical and structural terms: we say that it constitutes a superior dynamical unity.

New physics and new biomedicine gave us some crucial tools to transcend Descartes. The immense complexity and dimensionality of human systems, if considered in a post-Cartesian view, must be studied in the modern terms of complexity theory, nonlinear dynamics, field theory, quantum mechanics, molecular biology and cognitive science. These seemingly different approaches are integrated in order to reach a real view of MF nature and operations, beyond the dichotomies and appearances we are used to see.

A logical consequence is that MF, in its structure (that we recognize in networks) and dynamics (that we recognize in fields / waves of synchronizing nonlinear oscillators), would be heterogeneous. Dynamics, fields and the hyperstructure of MF would span through molecular domains, neural domains, cognitive domains and even socio-cultural domains. We need to consider how MF fields "pack" specific *synchronous dynamics* "vertically" ranging across these different domains, just as we have considered *diachronic dynamical fields* spanning "horizontally" within a single domain.

If we are able to accomplish this reframing of our perceptual and cognitive habits in order to recognize Mind Force, we might see how it forms a dynamical "glue" ensuring attractions in bodies, minds and social ensembles and the cohesion of our inner and outer bio-psychosocial realities. A definition of Mind Force would be as *the dynamical hyperstructure formed by networks of synchronized oscillators coupled in fields spanning trough heterogeneous domains* (Orsucci, 2009).

In conclusion, Mind Force theory is based on the integration of 4 main pillar-theories:

- Complexity theory
- Synchronization theory
- Network theory
- Field theory

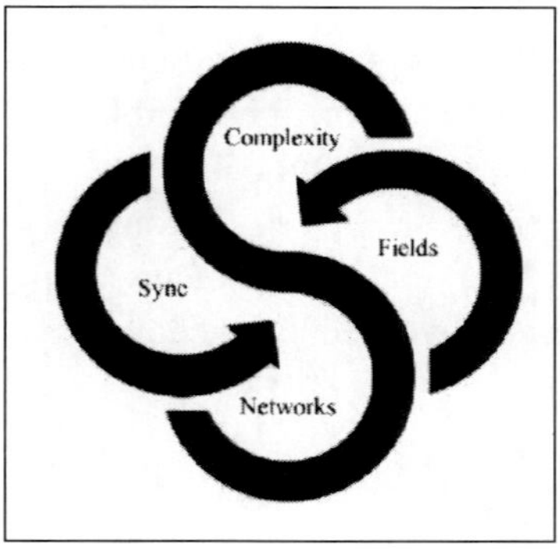

Figure 5. The four pillars of Mind Force.

Within the population of bio-psychosocial oscillators some act as master hubs, others as slave or free (Nicolis and Prigogine, 1977; Kauffman, 1993; 1995; 2000; Kelso, 1995) nodes within the MF hyperstructure dynamics. Waves of massive and heterogeneous transient entrainment would form attractors and fields. These waves of massive synchronizations propagate through different media, domains and scales. A logical consequence is that MF transient or steady fields interfere and interact, producing MF resultants, forming MF dynamical landscapes.

In conclusion, to use an expression coined by Douglas Hofstadter (2007: 39) Mind Force is the result of "the causal potency of collective phenomena" and patterns.

9. Modeling

The basic modeling for Mind Force is grounded in the network of oscillators' dynamics. To start, a pair of oscillators interacting through phase differences satisfies equations of the form

$$\theta_1' = \omega_1 + H_1(\theta_2 - \theta_1),$$
$$\theta_2' = \omega_2 + H_2(\theta_1 - \theta_2).$$

Here θ_i are the phases of the oscillators, ω_i are the frequencies of the uncoupled oscillators, and H_i are smooth 2π-periodic functions of the phase differences.

From a more abstract viewpoint, synchronization has been identified as a generic form of collective behavior in ensembles of dynamical systems with long range coupling. Several models that capture the essence of synchronization phenomena have been thoroughly studied over the last few decades. Kuramoto (1984) for instance, has analyzed an ensemble of N coupled phase oscillators, governed by the equations

$$\dot{\phi}_i(t) = \Omega_i + \frac{\varepsilon}{N}\sum_{j=1}^{N}\sin(\phi_j - \phi_i).$$

$i = 1,\ldots, N$, where $\varepsilon > 0$ is the strength of coupling. In the absence of coupling, $\varepsilon = 0$, each oscillator i performs a uniform angular motion with its natural frequency Ω_i. For $\varepsilon \neq 0$, the oscillators are globally coupled in the sense that the strength of the pair interaction does not depend on their relative position, but only on their relative state. In other words, each oscillator interacts with the rest of the system through global averages only.

Kuramoto has shown that, in the limit $N \to \infty$, there exists a critical value ε_c of the coupling intensity such that, for $\varepsilon > \varepsilon_c$, a subensemble of oscillators becomes entrained in periodic orbits with the same frequency, whereas the other oscillators remain unsynchronized.

A great deal of attention has been paid to the synchronization of ensembles formed by identical elements, especially, in the case where the individual dynamics is chaotic. Both continuous and discrete-time dynamics have been considered. Kaneko (1994) has introduced globally coupled chaotic maps as a mean-field model of lattice maps, which are extensively used to model complex extended systems (Kaneko, 1993).

For an ensemble of N maps whose individual dynamics is governed by the equation $w(t+1) = f[w(t)]$, global coupling is introduced as

$$\begin{aligned} \mathbf{w}_i(t+1) &= (1-\varepsilon)\mathbf{f}[\mathbf{w}_i(t)] + \frac{\varepsilon}{N}\sum_{j=1}^{N} \mathbf{f}[\mathbf{w}_j(t)] \\ &= (1-\varepsilon)\mathbf{f}[\mathbf{w}_i(t)] + \varepsilon\overline{\mathbf{f}(\mathbf{w})}, \end{aligned}$$

$i = 1,\ldots, N$, with $\varepsilon \in [0, 1]$. While for $\varepsilon = 0$ the elements evolve independently, for $\varepsilon = 1$ they become fully synchronized after the first time step.

Full synchronization is understood here as a situation where the individual states of all the elements in the ensemble coincide, i.e., where the trajectory of the system in phase space is restricted to the subspace $w_1 = w_2 = \ldots = w_N$. In this situation, the evolution of all the elements coincides with that of an independent element. The state of full synchronization can be asymptotically approached as the system evolves even for $\varepsilon < 1$. It has been shown that, if the individual dynamics is chaotic, full synchronization is linearly stable for $\varepsilon > \varepsilon_c$, where the critical value ε_c is related to the maximal Lyapunov exponent λ_M of the individual dynamics, as $\varepsilon_c = 1 - \exp(-\lambda_M)$. For nonchaotic individual dynamics where $\lambda_M < 0$, full synchronization is a stable state for any $\varepsilon > 0$. The connection between ε_c and λ_M makes it clear that the transition to full synchronization in chaotic systems, which has the character of a critical phenomenon, results from the competition between the stabilizing effect of global coupling and the inherent instability of chaotic orbits. Note carefully that the critical value ε_c does not depend on N, so that the synchronization threshold is the same for any size of the coupled ensemble.

For coupling strengths just below ε_c the system evolves asymptotically to a state of partial synchronization in the form of *clustering*, where the elements become divided into groups (Kaneko, 1989). Within each cluster the elements are fully synchronized but different clusters have different trajectories.

For large systems, the dynamics in the clustering regime is highly multistable and exhibits glassy-like features (Manrubia and Mikhailov, 2001).

In contrast with the critical value ε_c, the stability properties of the clustering regime are strongly dependent on the system size (Abramson, 2000).

Cross-Coupled Extended Systems provide a versatile collection of models for a wide class of complex natural phenomena, ranging from pattern formation in physicochemical reactions, to biological morphogenesis, to evolutionary processes.

It is therefore interesting to consider how these systems behave under the effect of mutual interactions and, in particular, study the synchronization properties of their coevolution when they are mutually coupled by algorithms similar to the scheme of coupling already presented (Zanette and Morelli, 2003).

P. M. Gleiser and D. H. Zanette (2006) analyzed the interplay of synchronization and structure evolution in an evolving network of phase oscillators. An initially random network is adaptively rewired according to the dynamical coherence of the oscillators, in order to enhance their mutual synchronization. They showed that the evolving network reaches a small-world structure. Its clustering coefficient attains a maximum for an intermediate intensity of the coupling between oscillators, where a rich diversity of synchronized oscillator groups is observed. In the stationary state, these synchronized groups are directly associated with network clusters.

Their model consists of an ensemble of N coupled phase oscillators, whose individual evolution is given by

$$\dot{\phi}_i = \omega_i + \frac{r}{M_i}\sum_{j=1}^{N} W_{ij}\sin(\phi_j - \phi_i),$$

$i = 1,\ldots,N$, where ω_i is the natural frequency of oscillator I and r is the coupling strength. The weights W_{ij} define the adjacency matrix of the interaction network: $W_{ij} = 1$ if oscillator i interacts with oscillator j, and 0 otherwise. The number of neighbors of oscillator i is $M_{ij} = \Sigma_j W_{ij}$. The adjacent matrix is symmetric, $W_{ij} = W_{ji}$, so that the network is a non directed graph.

Conclusion

A definition of Mind Force would be as the dynamical hyperstructure formed by networks of synchronized oscillators coupled in fields spanning trough heterogeneous domains. Mind Force theory is based on the integration of 4 main pillar-theories: Complexity theory; Synchronization theory; Network theory; Field theory. Mind Force is the result of the causal power of collective phenomena and patterns. The new theory of Mind Force represents an integration of different biophysical and cognitive domains considered as components of a dynamical hyper-network.

It can produce breakthrough advancements in consciousness studies, psychosocial and clinical applications. It might lead to new pathways in science and epistemology.

References

Abraham, F. D., Abraham, R., and Shaw, C. D. (1990). *A Visual Introduction To Dynamical Systems Theory For Psychology.* Santa Cruz, CA: Aerial Press.

Abramson, G. (2000) Long transients and cluster size in globally coupled maps, *Europhys. Lett.* 52(6), 615-619.

Aiello, L. C., and Wheeler, P. (1995). The expensive-tissue hypothesis. *Current Anthropology* 36:199 –221.

Ainsworth, M. D. (1969). Object relations, dependency, and attachment: a theoretical review of the infant-mother relationship. *Child Dev.,* 40, 969-1025.

Ainsworth, M. D. (1985). Attachments across the life span. *Bull. N. Y. Acad. Med.*, 61, 792-812.

Albert, R. and Barabasi, A. L. (2002) Statistical mechanics of complex networks, *Reviews Of Modern Physics,* Volume 74.

Ambrose, S. H. (2001). Paleolithic Technology and Human Evolution. *Science* 291, 1748-1753.

Amit, D. J. (1989). *Modeling Brain Function: The World Of Attractor Neural Networks*. New York, NY: Cambridge University Press.

Andrew, TJ, Purves D (2005) The wagon wheel illusion in continuous light, *Trends in Cog Neurosci* 9(6): 261-263.

Aoki, K., and Feldman M. V. (1987). Toward a theory for the evolution of culture, *Proceedings of the National Academy of Sciences USA* 84:7164 – 68.

Arbib, M. A. and Mundhenk, T. N. (2005). Schizophrenia and the mirror system: an essay. *Neuropsychologia,* 43, 268-280.

Arbib, M. A. (2001). Co-evolution of human consciousness and language. *Ann. N. Y. Acad. Sci.*, 929, 195-220.

Arbib, M. A. (2002). The Mirror System, Imitation, and the Evolution of Language, in *Imitation in Animals and Artifacts,* (Chrystopher Nehaniv and Kerstin Dautenhahn, Editors), The MIT Press.

Arbib, M. A. (2005). From monkey-like action recognition to human language: an evolutionary framework for neurolinguistics. *Behav. Brain Sci.,* 28, 105-124.

Arbib, M. A. (2007). Other faces in the mirror: a perspective on schizophrenia. *World Psychiatry,* 6, 11-14.

Ashby, W. R. (1952) *Design for a Brain*, London: Chapman and Hall.

Atmanspacher, H. (2004) Quantum theory and consciousness: an overview with selected examples, *Discrete Dynamics in Nature and Society*, 1, 51-73.

Austin, J. H. (2006) *Zen-Brain Reflections*, Cambridge: MIT press.

Baer, R. A. (2003). Mindfulness Training as a Clinical Intervention: A Conceptual and Empirical Review. *Clinical Psychology: Science and Practice*, 10, 125-143.

Bak, P., Tang, C., Wiesenfeld, K. (1984) Self-organized criticality: an explanation of 1/f noise, *Physical Review Letters,* 59:381-384.

Bak, P. (1990) Simulation of self-organized criticality, *Physica Scripta,* T33.

Bak P. (1996). *How Nature Works, The Science Of Self-Organized Criticality*, New York, NY, USA: Copernicus.

Barabasi, A.-L. and Albert, R. (1999) Emergence of scaling in random networks. *Science* 286, 509–512.

Barabasi, A.-L. (2005) Taming complexity, *Nature,* 1: 68-70.

Barahona, M., Pecora, L. M. (2002) Synchronization in Small-World Systems *Physical Review Letters, 89, 054101*

Bartels, A. and Zeki, S. (2000) The neural basis of romantic love, *Neuroreport*, 11(17):3829-3834.

Bates, E. (1979). *The Emergence Of Symbols, Cognition And Communication In Infancy,* New York: Academic Press.

Bates, E. and MacWhinney, B. (1987). Competition, variation and language learning. MacWhinney, B. (ed.). *Mechanisms of Language Acquisition*, (pp. 157-193) Hillsdale, NJ: Erlbaum.

Bateson, G. (1987*). Steps To An Ecology Of Mind, Collected Essays In Anthropology, Psychiatry, Evolution, And Epistemology*, Northvale, N.J: Aronson.

Bergson, H. B. (1911). *Creative Evolution* tr. Arthur Mitchell, Henry Holt and Company.

Bion, W. R. (1992). *Cogitations*, London: Karnac Books.

Boccaletti, S., Grebogi, C., Lai, Y.-C., Mancini, H., and Maza, D. (2000). The control of chaos: theory and applications. *Physics Reports* 329[3], 103-197.

Boccaletti, S., Pecora, L. M., and Pelaez, A. (2001). Unifying framework for synchronization of coupled dynamical systems. *Phys. Rev. E.*, 63, 066219.

Bodmer, W. F. and Cavalli-Sforza, L. L. (1976). *Genetics, evolution and man*, San Francisco: Freeman.

Bohm, D. and Hiley, B. J. (2008). *The Undivided Universe*. London: Routledge.

Borges J. L. (1964) *Labyrinths, Selected Stories and Other Writings*, New York: New Directions Pub. Corp.

Bowlby, J. (1978). Attachment theory and its therapeutic implications. *Adolesc. Psychiatry*, 6, 5-33.

Bowlby, J. (1982). Attachment and loss: retrospect and prospect. *Am. J. Orthopsychiatry*, 52, 664-678.

Boyd, R. and Richerson, P. J. (1985) *Culture and the Evolutionary Process*. Chicago: University of Chicago Press.

Branigan, H. P., Pickering, M. J. and Cleland, A. A. (2000). Syntactic co-ordination in dialogue. *Cognition*, 75, B13-25.

Breuer, J. and Freud, S. (1895). *Studien über Hysterie.* Leipzig: F. Deuticke.

Cancedda L., Putignano E, Sale A, Viegi A, Berardi N, and Maffei L (2004) Acceleration of Visual System Development by Environmental Enrichment, *J. Neurosci.*, 24: 4840 - 4848.

Canetti, E. (1962) *Crowds And Power*, London: Gollancz.

Carbonara, D. (ed.) (2005). *Technology Literacy Applications in Learning Environments*, Hersey, NJ: Idea Group.

Carroll, T. L. and Pecora, L. M. (1993a) Stochastic resonance and crises, *Physical Review Letters*, 70, 576-579.

Carroll, T. L. and Pecora, L. M. (1993b) Using chaos to keep period-multiplied systems in phase, *Physical Review E*. 48, 2426-2436.

Chalmers, D. J. (1995) *Explaining Consciousness: The Hard Problem*. MIT Press.

Chalmers, D. J. (1996) *The Conscious Mind. In Search of a Fundamental Theory*. Oxford: Oxford University Press.

Chan, P. A., and Rabinowitz, T. (2006). A cross-sectional analysis of video games and attention deficit hyperactivity disorder symptoms in adolescents, *Ann Gen Psychiatry*. Oct 24; 5:16.

Changeux, J.-P. (2004). *The Physiology of Truth: Neuroscience and Human Knowledge.* Harvard University Press.

Chomsky, N. (1975). *Reflections on Language.* New York: Pantheon,

Chomsky, N. (1993). *Language And Thought.* (1st ed.) Wakefield, R. I: Moyer Bell.

Churchland, P. M. (1995). The puzzle of conscious experience. *Scientific American* 273, 80–86.

Corrao, F. (1986). Il concetto di campo come modello teorico, in *Gruppo e Funzione analitica*, VII, N. 1.

Corrao, F. (1992). *Modelli Psicoanalitici. Mito, Passione, Memoria*. Bari: Editori Laterza.

Crick, F. and Koch, C. (2003). A framework for consciousness, *Nature Neuroscience*, 6-2.

Crutchfield, J. P. and Kaneko, K. (1987) Phenomenology of Spatiotemporal Chaos, in *Directions in Chaos*, World Scientific, 272-353.

Dale, R., and Spivey, M. J. (2006). Unraveling the dyad: Using recurrence analysis to explore patterns of syntactic coordination between children and caregivers in conversation. *Language Learning*, 56, 391-430.

Damasio, A. R. (1998a). Emotion in the perspective of an integrated nervous system. *Brain Res. Rev.*, 26, 83-86.

Damasio, A. R. (1998b). Investigating the biology of consciousness. *Philos. Trans. R. Soc. Lond. B Biol. Sci.*, 353, 1879-1882.

Damasio, A. R. (1999). How the brain creates the mind. *Sci. Am.*, 281, 112-117.

Darwin, C. R. (1909). *The Origin Of Species.* New York: P. F. Collier and son.

Dawkins, R. (1976). *The Selfish Gene,* Oxford: Oxford University Press.

Dawkins, R. (1982). *The Extended Phenotype.* San Francisco, CA: Freeman.

De Risio, S. and Orsucci, F. (2004). *Bioethics In Complexity, Foundations And Evolutions.* London: Imperial College Press.

Dennett, D. C. (1991). *Consciousness explained,* Boston: Little, Brown and Co.

Descartes, R. (1988). *The Philosophical Writings Of Descartes*, Cambridge: Cambridge University Press.
Donald, M. (1997). Origins of the modern mind: Three stages in the evolution of culture and cognition. *Behavioral and Brain Sciences* 16 (4): 737-791.
Dubé, J. and Desprès, P. (2000). The Control of Dynamical Systems - Recovering Order from Chaos. In Y. Itikawa (Ed.), *The Physics of Electronic and Atomic Collisions*, Woodbury, N.Y.: AIP.
Eccles, J. C. (1990). A unitary hypothesis of mind–brain interaction in cerebral cortex. *Proc. R. Soc., London B* 240, 433–451.
Eckmann, J-P., Kamphorst, S. O., and Ruelle, D. (1987). Recurrence plots of dynamical systems, *Europhysics Letters*, 5, 973-977.
Eco, U. (1989). *The open work*. Cambridge, Mass: Harvard University Press.
Eco, U. (1990). *The limits of interpretation*. Bloomington, Ind: Indiana University Press.
Edelman, G. M. (1989) *Neural Darwinism: The Theory of Neuronal Group Selection*. New York: Basic Books.
Edelman, G. M. and Tononi G. (2000). *A Universe Of Consciousness. How Matter Becomes Imagination*. New York, NY: Basic Books.
Edwards, J. C. W. (2005). Is Consciousness Only a Property of Individual Cells? *Journal of Consciousness Studies,* 12.
Eliasmith, C. (2005). A unified approach to building and controlling spiking attractor networks. *Neural Computation*. 17(6): 1276-1314
Ellenberger, H. F. (1970). *The Discovery Of The Unconscious. The History And Evolution Of Dynamic Psychiatry*. New York: Basic Books.
Beck F., Eccles J. (1992). Quantum Aspects of Brain Activty and the Role of Consciousness, *Proc. Nat. Acad. Sci. USA*, 89: 11357-11361.
Feldman, M. W., and Laland, K. N. (1996). Gene-culture coevolutionary theory, *Trends in Ecology and Evolution* 11:453 – 457.
Fisher H. E., Aron A., Mashek D., Li H., Brown L. L. (2002) Defining the Brain Systems of Lust, Romantic Attraction, and Attachment - *Archives of Sexual Behavior*, Vol. 31, No. 5.
Fonagy, P. and Target, M. (1997). Attachment and reflective function: Their role in self-organization, *Development and Psychopathology*, 9 679–700.
Fonagy P. (2002). *Affect Regulation, Mentalization, and The Development Of The Self*. New York: Other Press.
Freeman, W. J. (1975). *Mass Action In The Nervous System*, NY, Academic Press.
Freeman, W. J. (1978). Spatial properties of an EEG event in the olfactory bulb and cortex. *Electroencephalogr. Clin. Neurophysiol.,* 44, 586-605.
Freeman, W. J. (1997). Neurohumoral brain dynamics of social group formation. Implications for autism. *Ann. N. Y. Acad. Sci.,* 807, 501-503.
Freeman, W. J. (1999). *How brains make up their minds*. London: Weidenfeld and Nicolson.
Freeman, W. J. (2000). Mesoscopic neurodynamics: from neuron to brain. *J. Physiol Paris*, 94, 303-322.
Freeman, W. J. (2006). A cinematographic hypothesis of cortical dynamics in perception. *Int. J. Psychophysiol.*, 60, 149-161.

Freeman, W. J. (2007). Indirect biological measures of consciousness from field studies of brains as dynamical systems. *Neural Netw.,* 20, 1021-1031.

Freeman, W. J., and Vitiello, G. (2006). Nonlinear brain dynamics as macroscopic manifestation of underlying many-body field dynamics. *Physics of Life Reviews*, 3, 93–118.

Freud, S. (1959) *Collected Papers*, New York: Basic Books.

Freud, S. (1985) *The Complete Letters Of Sigmund Freud To Wilhelm Fliess,* 1887-1904, Cambridge, Mass: Belknap Press.

Gaddini, E. (1969). On Imitation. *Int. J. Psycho-Anal.,* 50:475-484.

Gaddini, E., (1989). *Scritti, 1953-1985.* Milano: R. Cortina.

Gazzaniga, M. S. (2005). *The Ethical Brain.* New York: The Dana Press.

Gibson, J. J. (1979). *The Ecological Approach To Visual Perception.* Boston: Houghton Mifflin.

Gleiser, P. M. and Zanette, D. H. (2006) Synchronization and structure in an adaptive oscillator network, *Eur. Phys. J. B* 53, 233–238.

Goleman, D. (1977) *The Varieties Of The Meditative Experience*, New York: Irvington Publishers.

Goleman, D. (1995). *Emotional Intelligence*, New York: Bantam Books.

Green, C. S., and Bavelier D. (2003). Action video game modifies visual selective attention. *Nature,* Vol 423, 534-537.

Groddeck, G., and Freud, S. (1970). *Der Mensch und sein Es. Briefe, Aufs tue, Biografisches*,[*Man and his It. Letters, essays, biographical*] Wiesbaden: Limes Verlag.

Grush, R. and Churchland, P. (1995) Gap's in Penrose's Toilings*, Journal of Consciousness Studies,* 2(1), pp. 10-29.

Hagan, S., Hameroff, S. and Tuszynski, J. (2002) Quantum computation in brain microtubules? Decoherence and biological feasibility, *Physical Reviews E,* 65.

Haken, H. and Stadler, M. (1990). *Synergetics Of Cognition*, Berlin: Springer-Verlag.

Haken, H. and Mikhailov, A. S. (1993). *Interdisciplinary approaches to nonlinear complex systems*. Berlin: Springer-Verlag.

Hall, E. T. (1983). *The Dance of Life: The Other Dimension of Time.* New York: Anchor Press/Doubleday.

Hameroff, S. (1987) *Ultimate Computing,* Elsevier.

Hameroff, S. (2006). Consciousness, neurobiology and quantum mechanics, In: *The Emerging Physics of Consciousness*, (Ed.) Tuszynski, J. NY: Elsevier.

Hebb, D. O. (1949). *The Organization Of Behavior*. New York, NY: Wiley.

Hofer, M. A. (1984). Relationships as regulators: a psychobiologic perspective on bereavement. *Psychosom. Med.,* 46, 183-197.

Hofer, M. A. (1994a). Early relationships as regulators of infant physiology and behavior. *Acta Paediatr. Suppl,* 397, 9-18.

Hofer, M. A. (1994b). Hidden regulators in attachment, separation, and loss. *Monogr. Soc. Res. Child Dev.,* 59, 192-207.

Hofstadter, D. (2007). *I Am A Strange Loop*. New York: Basic Books.

Hopfield, J. J. (1982). Neural networks and physical systems with emergent collective computational abilities. *Proceedings of the National Academy of Sciences* 79, 2554–2558.

Hume, D. (1854). *The Philosophical Works Of David Hume*. Boston: Little, Brown and Company.

Husserl, E. (1980). *Collected Works,* Boston: The Hague.

Insel, T. R., Young, L., Wang, Z. (1997) Molecular aspects of monogamy. *Ann N Y Acad Sci.* Jan 15;807:302-16.

Jacob, S. and McClintock, M. K. (2000). Psychological state and mood effects of steroidal chemosignals in women and men. *Horm. Behav.,* 37, 57-78.

James, W. (1967). *The Writings Of William James* (McDermott JJ ed) New York; Random House.

Jones, F. J. (1995). *The structure of Petrarch's Canzoniere*. Cambridge: Brewer.

Jourdain, R. (1997). *Music, The Brain, And Ecstasy: How Music Captures Our Imagination.* New York: Harper Perennial.

Jung, C. G. and Pauli, W. (1955). *The Interpretation of Nature and the Psyche*. NY: Pantheon Books.

Kandel, E. R. (1999). Biology and the Future of Psychoanalysis: A New Intellectual Framework for Psychiatry Revisited, *Am J Psychiatry* 156: 505-524.

Kaneko, K. (1993) *Theory And Applications Of Coupled Map Lattices*. Chichester: Wiley.

Kaneko, K. (1994) Relevance of clustering to biological networks, *Physica D,* 75(1-3), 55-73.

Kauffman, S. A. (1993). *The Origins Of Order, Self Organization And Selection In Evolution,* New York: Oxford University Press.

Kauffman, S. A. (1995). *At Home In The Universe. The Search For Laws Of Self-Organization And Complexity,* New York: Oxford University Press.

Kauffman, S. A. (2000). *Investigations.* Oxford: Oxford University Press.

Kelso, J. A. S. and Clark, J. E. (1982). *The Development Of Movement Control And Coordination.* Chichester West Sussex: Wiley.

Kelso, J. A. S., Mandell, A. J., Shlesinger, M. F., Haken, H. (1988). *Dynamic Patterns In Complex Systems.* Singapore: World Scientific.

Kelso J. A. S. (1995). *Dynamic Patterns, The Self-Organization Of Brain And Behavior,* Cambridge, Mass: MIT Press.

Kernberg, P. F. (2007). *Beyond the Reflection: The Role of the Mirror Paradigm in Clinical Practice,* New York: Other Press.

Kornhuber, H. H., Deecke, L. (1965). Hirnpotentialänderungen bei Willkürbewegungen und passiven Bewegungen des Menschen: Bereitschaftspotential und Reafferente Potentiale.[Brain potential changes in voluntary and passive human movements: readiness potential and reafferent potentials] *Pflügers Arch. ges. Physiol.* 284 1-17.

Kozma, R. and Freeman, W. J. (2003). Basic principles of the KIV model and its application to the navigation problem. *J. Integr. Neurosci.,* 2, 125-145.

Kozma, R., Puljic, M., Balister, P., Bollobas, B., and Freeman, W. J. (2005). Phase transitions in the neuropercolation model of neural populations with mixed local and non-local interactions. *Biol. Cybern.,* 92, 367-379.

Kupfer, D. J., Monk, T. H., Barchas, J. D. (1988). *Biological Rhythms And Mental Disorders.* New York: Guilford Press.

Lacan, J. (1937). *Ecrits.* New York: W. W. Norton (New Ed edition 2005).

LaForge, R. (2004). The Early Development of the Interpersonal System of Personality (ISP), *Multivariate Behavioral Research,* Volume 39, Issue 2, pages 359 – 378.

Laland, K. N., Odling-Smee, J., and Feldman, M. W. (2000). Niche construction, biological evolution, and cultural change, *Behavioral And Brain Sciences* 23, 131–175.

LeDoux J. E. (2002). *Synaptic Self, How Our Brains Become Who We Are*. New York: Viking.

Leibniz, G. W. (1996). *New Essays On Human Understanding*. Cambridge: Cambridge University Press.

Lewin, K. (May, 1939) Field Theory and Experiment in Social Psychology: Concepts and Methods, *The American Journal of Sociology*, Vol. 44, No. 6, pp. 868-896.

Lewin, K. (1943) Psychological ecology, in: D. Cartwright (Ed.) (1952) *Field Theory in Social Science, Social Science,* Paperbacks, London.

Lewontin, R. C. (1983). Gene, organism, and environment. In: *Evolution From Molecules To Men,* ed. D. S. Bendall. Cambridge University Press.

Libet, B. (1993). *Neurophysiology Of Consciousness: Selected Papers And New Essays*, Boston: Birkhauser.

Libet, B. (1994). A testable field theory of the mind-brain interaction, *J. Consciousness Stud.* 1, 119-126.

Libet, B. J. (1996) Conscious Mind as a Field, *J. Theor. Biol.* 178, 223-2243.

Libet, B. J. (1997). Conscious Mind as a Force Field: A Reply to Lindahl and Arhem, *J. Theor. Biol.* 185, 137-138.

Libet, B. J., Freeman, A., and Sutherland, K. (1999). *The Volitional Brain, Towards A Neuroscience Of Free Will,* Thorverton, UK: Imprint Academic.

Libet, B. J. (2006). Reflections on the interaction of the mind and brain, *Progress in Neurobiology,* 78, 322–326.

Lieberman, P. (1991). *Uniquely Human: The Evolution of Speech, Thought, and Selfless Behavior.* Harvard University Press, Cambridge, Massachusetts.

Lindahl, B. I. and Arhem, P. (1994). Mind as a force field: comments on a new interactionistic hypothesis. *J. Theor. Biol.*, 171, 111-122.

Lindahl, B. I. and Arhem, P. (1996). The mental force field hypothesis: a reply to Libet. *J. theor. Biol.* 178, 225-226.

Lorenz, E. N. (1993). *The Essence Of Chaos.* Seattle: University of Washington Press.

Lorenzana, Alvarez de, J. M., Ward, L. M. (1987) On evolutionary systems, *Behav Sci.* Jan;32(1):19-33.

Margenau, H. (1984). *The Miracle of Existence,* Woodbridge, Conn.: Ox Bow Press.

Marwan, N. (2003). *Encounters With Neighbours,* doctoral dissertation, University of Potsdam.

Mathiak, K., Weber, R. (2006). Toward brain correlates of natural behavior: fMRI during violent video games. *Hum Brain Mapp.* Dec;27(12):948-956.

Maturana, H. R., and Varela, F. J. (1980). *Autopoiesis And Cognition, The Realization Of The Living.* Dordrecht, Holland: D. Reidel Pub. Co.

Maturana, H. (2002). Autopoiesis, Structural Coupling and Cognition: A history of these and other notions in the biology of cognition. *Cybernetics and Human Knowing* 9 (3-4): 5-34.

McClintock, M. K., Bullivant, S., Jacob, S., Spencer, N., Zelano, B., and Ober, C. (2005). Human body scents: conscious perceptions and biological effects. *Chem. Senses*, 30 Suppl 1, i135-i137.

Mittag, M., Volker W. (2003). The circadian clock of the unicellular eukaryotic model organism Chlamydomonas reinhardtii, *Biological Chemistry,* vol. 384, no5, pp. 689-695.

Neri C. (1993). Campo. *Psiche,* Anno 1, n. 2, 1993, 289-295.

Neri, C. (1998). *Group.* London: Jessica Kingsley.

Nishikawa, T., Motter, A. E., Lai, Y. C., Hoppensteadt, F. C. (2003). Heterogeneity in Oscillator Networks: Are Smaller Worlds Easier to Synchronize, *Physical Review Letters.*

Norman, D. A. (1988). *The Design of Everyday Things.* New York: Doubleday.

Norman, D. A. (1999). Affordances, Conventions, and Design, *Interactions,* 6 (3) p. 38-41.

Orsucci, F. (1996a). Chaos and complexity in psychopathology. *Giorn. Ital. Psicopat.*, 3.

Orsucci, F. (1996b). Behcet's disease and psychosomatic patterns of thinking. A single case study. *Psychother. Psychosom.,* 65, 112-114.

Orsucci, F., (ed) (1998). *The Complex Matters Of The Mind*, Singapore: World Scientific.

Orsucci, F., Walters, K., Giuliani, A., Webber, Jr C., and Zbilut, J. (1999). Orthographic Structuring of Human Speech and Texts, *International Journal of Chaos Theory and Applications,* Vol. 4-2, pp. 80-88.

Orsucci, F. (2000). Olfaction: New Frontiers for Cognitive Sciences. (Edited by C Di Natale, A D'Amico and P Siciliano). *Sensors and Microsystems*, Singapore: World Scientific Publishing.

Orsucci, F. (2002a). Linguistic landscapes. *Chaos and Complexity Letters,* 1, 2.

Orsucci, F. (2002b). *Changing Mind*, Singapore: World Scientific.

Orsucci, F., Giuliani, A., Zbilut. J., (2004). Structure and Coupling of Semiotic Sets, *Experimental Chaos*, American Institute of Physics, *AIP Proceedings*, Vol. 742, pp. 83-93.

Orsucci, F., and Sala, N. (2005). Virtual Reality, Telemedicine and Beyond. (Carbonara, D. ed.). *Technology Literacy Applications in Learning Environments.* (pp. 349-357) Idea Group, Hersey.

Orsucci, F., Giuliani, A., Webber, C., Zbilut, J., Fonagy, P., and Mazza, M., (2006) Combinatorics and synchronization in natural semiotics, *Physica A: Statistical Mechanics and its Applications* – Elsevier 361: 665–676.

Orsucci, F. and Sala, N. (2006). *New Research on Chaos And Complexity.* New York: Nova Science Publishers.

Orsucci, F. (2006). The paradigm of complexity in clinical neuro-cognitive science. *The Neuroscientist* – SAGE, Vol. 12- 4, 1-10.

Orsucci, F. (2009) Mind Force, modeling a biophysical hyperstructure, *Chaos and Complexity Letters,* 4-1.

Ott, E. Grebogi C. and Yorke, J. A. (1990) Controlling chaos, *Phvsical Review Letters*, vol. 64. no. 11, pp. 1196-1199.

Paetkau, V., Roderic, E., and Reinhard. I. (2006). A model for generating circadian rhythm by coupling ultradian oscillators, *Theoretical Biology and Medical Modelling,* 3:12.

Paley, B (2002) *TextArc* - extracting new meaning and relationships from literary works - new visual cataloguing approach, http://www.textarc.org/.

Palla, G., Barabasi, A.-L., and Vicsek, T. (2007) Quantifying social group evolution, *Nature*, Vol 446.

Panksepp, J. (1998). *Affective Neuroscience, the Foundations of Human and Animal Emotions*, New York: Oxford University Press.

Panksepp, J. (2004). *Textbook of Biological Psychiatry*. Hoboken, N.J: Wiley-Liss.

Pecora, L. M. and Carroll, T. L. (1990). Synchronization in chaotic systems. *Physical Review Letters,* 64, 821-824.

Pecora, L. M. and Carroll, T. L. (1991). Driving systems with chaotic signals. *Physical Review A*, 44, 2374-2383.

Pecora, L. M. and Barahona, M. (2008) Synchronization of oscillators in complex networks, *Pramana*, Vol. 70, No. 6.

Peirce, C. S. (1931). *Collected papers of Charles Sanders Peirce.* Cambridge: Harvard University Press.

Penrose, R. (1989). *The Emperor's New Mind,* Oxford: Oxford University Press.

Penrose, R. (1994). *Shadows of the Mind,* Oxford: Oxford University Press.

Petitot, J. (1999). *Naturalizing Phenomenology, Issues In Contemporary Phenomenology And Cognitive Science*, Stanford Ca: Stanford University Press.

Piaget, J. (1930). *The child's conception of physical causality.* London: Kegan Paul, Trench, and Trubner. (Original work published in French in 1927).

Popper, K. R. (1993) A discussion on the mind-body problem, *Theor. Med.* 14, 167-180.

Porphyry of Tyre (1940) *Isagoge,* in Catalogus Codicum astrologorum Graecorum, Stefan Weinstock, ed. Franz Cumon, ed. (Brussels,): V.4, 187-228.

Port, R., Tajima, K., and Cummins, F. (1999). *Non-linear Analysis of Developmental Processes* (van der Maas and van Geert ed), Amsterdam, NE: Elsevier.

Pribram, K. (1971). *Languages of the Brain*, Prentice-Hall, New Jersey.

Purves, D (2003) *Why We See What We Do: An Empirical Theory of Vision*, Sinauer Associates, Inc.

Pyragas, K. (1996). Weak and strong synchronization of chaos. *Physical.Review.E.*, 54, R4508-R4511.

Pyragas, K. (2001). Control of chaos via an unstable delayed feedback controller. *Phys.Rev.Lett.,* 86, 2265-2268.

Quillian, M. R. (1967), Word Concepts: A Theory and Simulation of Some Basic Semantic Capabilities, *Behavioral Science* 12: 410-430.

Quintero, J. E., Kuhlman, S. J. and McMahon, D. G. (2003) The Biological Clock Nucleus: A Multiphasic Oscillator Network Regulated by Light, *The Journal of Neuroscience,* September 3, 23(22):8070-8076.

Reppert, S.M., Weaver, D. R. (2002) Coordination of circadian timing in mammals, *Nature,* 418, 6901, pp. 935-941

Ricciardi, L. M. and Umezawa, H. (1967). Brain and physics of many-body problems. *Kybernetik,* 4, 44-48.

Richards, G. (1997). *Race, racism, and psychology: Towards a reflexive history*. New York: Routledge.

Richardson, D.C., and Dale, R. (2005). Looking to understand: The coupling between speakers' and listeners' eye movements and its relationship to discourse comprehension. *Cognitive Science,* 29, 39-54.

Rinaldi, S. (1998b). Laura and Petrarch: An intriguing case of cyclical love dynamics. SIAM *Journal on Applied Mathematics,* 58, 1205-1221.

Rizzolatti, G., and Arbib, M.A. (1998). Language within our grasp. *Trends in Neuroscience* 21, 188-194. Vintage Books ed., rev. and expanded ed.) New York: Vintage Books.

Rossi, E. L. (1996) The psychobiology of mind-body communication: The complex, self-organizing field of information transduction, *BioSystems* 38, 199-206.

Sacks, O. W. (2004). In the River of Consciousness *The New York Review of Books*: volume 51, number 1.

Sacks, O. W. (2007). *Musicophilia, Tales of Music and the Brain,* New York: Alfred A. Knopf.

Sale A, Putignano E, Cancedda L, Landia S, Cirulli F, Berardi N, and Maffei L, (2004) Enriched environment and acceleration of visual system development, *Neuropharmacology*, 47, 5, 649-660.

Schopen, A. and Freeman, B. (1992) Meditation: The Forgotten Western Tradition. *Counseling and Values*, v36 n2 p123-34.

Shockley, K., Santana, M. V., and Fowler, C. A. (2003). Mutual interpersonal postural constraints are involved in cooperative conversation. *Journal of Experimental Psychology: Human Perception and Performance,* 29, 326-332.

Siegel, D.J. (2007). *The Mindful Brain,* New York: Norton.

Skarda, C. A. and Freeman W. J., (1987) How Brains Make Chaos in Order to Make Sense of the World, *Behavioral and Brain Sciences,* 2, 10.

Somers, D. and Kopell, N. (1995) Waves and synchrony in networks of oscillators of relaxation and non-relaxation type, *Physica D* 89 169-183.

Sperry, R. W. (1947) Cerebral regulation of motor coordination in monkeys following multiple transections of sensorimotor cortex, *J Neurophysiol*, 10, 275-294.

Sperry, R.W. (1980). Mind–brain interaction: mentalism, yes; dualism, no. *Neuroscience* 5, 195–206.

Stapp, H. P. (1993) A quantum theory of the mind-brain interface, in *Mind, Matter, and Quantum Mechanics*, Springer-Verlag, Berlin, pp. 145–172.

Stern, D. (1985). *The Interpersonal World Of The Infant*. New York: Basic Books.

Stern, D. N. (2004). *The Present Moment In Psychotherapy And Everyday Life.* New York: W.W. Norton.

Stern, K. and McClintock, M. K. (1998). Regulation of ovulation by human pheromones. *Nature,* 392, 177-179.

Stewart, J. and Varela, F. J. (1991). Morphogenesis in shape-space. Elementary meta-dynamics in a model of the immune network. *J.Theor.Biol.,* 153, 477-498.

Straker, L.M., Pollock, C.M., Zubrick, S.R., and Kurinczuk, J.J. (2006). The association between information and communication technology exposure and physical activity, musculoskeletal and visual symptoms and socio-economic status in 5-year-olds. *Child Care Health Dev.* 32(3): 343-51.

Strogatz, S. H. (1994). *Nonlinear Dynamics and Chaos: With Applications to Physics, Biology, Chemistry, and Engineering*. Reading, MA: Addison-Wesley.

Strogatz, S. H. (2003). *Sync. The Emerging Science of Spontaneous Order*. New York: Hyperion.

Tegmark, M. (2000) Importance of quantum coherence in brain processes, *Physical Reviews E*, 61, pp. 4194-4206.

Thompson, E. and Varela, F. J. (2001). Radical embodiment: neural dynamics and consciousness. *Trends Cogn Sci.,* 5, 418-425.

Thompson, W.I. (1996). Coming Into Being: Artifacts And Texts In The Evolution Of Consciousness. New York: St. Martin's Press.

Tomasello, M. (2003). *A Usage-Based Theory of Language*, Cambridge, MA: Harvard University Press.

Tsuda, I. (2001). Toward an interpretation of dynamic neural activity in terms of chaotic dynamical systems. *Behavioral Brain Ssciences* 24 (5): 793-810.

Turing, A. M. (1996). *The legacy of Alan Turing.* Oxford: Clarendon Press.

Umezawa, H. and Vitiello, G. (1986) *Quantum Mechanics,* Napoli: Bibliopolis.

van Gelder, T. (1998). The dynamical hypothesis in cognitive science. *Behavioral and Brain Sciences,*

Varela, F.J., Thompson, E., Rosch, E. (1991). *The Embodied Mind, Cognitive Science And Human Experience,* Cambridge, Mass: MIT Press.

Varela, F. J. (1999). Cognition without representations. *Riv. Biol.,* 92, 511-512.

Varela, F. J., Lachaux, J. P., Rodriguez, E., and Martinerie J. (2001). The brainweb: phase synchronization and large-scale integration. *Nat.Rev.Neurosci.* 2 (4): 229-239.

Verhulst, F. (1994). Metaphors for psychoanalysis. *Nonlinear Science Today,* 4, 1-6.

Vitiello, G. (1995). Dissipation and memory capacity in the quantum brain model, *Internat. J. Modern Phys. B* 9 973–989.

Vitiello, G. (2001) *My Double Unveiled: The Dissipative Quantum Model of the Brain.* Amsterdam: John Benjamins.

Vitiello, G. (2002). *Dissipative quantum brain dynamics, No Matter, Never Mind* (K. Yasue, M. Jibu, and T. Della Senta, eds.), Amsterdam: John Benjamins, pp. 43–61.

von Neumann, J. (2004). *Mathematical Foundations of Quantum Mechanics*. Princeton University Press, 11:3829–34.

Ward, L. M. (2002). *Dynamical Cognitive Science.* Cambridge, Mass: MIT Press.

Watts, D.J., Strogatz, S. H. (1998) Collective dynamics of 'small-world' networks. *Nature.* Jun 4;393(6684):409-10.

Webber, C.L. Jr, and Zbilut, J.P. (1994). Dynamical assessment of physiological systems and states using recurrence plot strategies, *Journal of Applied Physiology,* 76, 965-973.

Welsh, D. K. (1995) Individual neurons dissociated from rat suprachiasmatic nucleus express independently phased circadian firing rhythms, *Neuron,* Vol. 14,697-706.

West, B. J. (2006). *Where Medicine Went Wrong, Rediscovering The Path To Complexity*. New Jersey: World Scientific.

Whitehead, A. N. (1978). *Process and Reality.* New York: The Free Press.

Wiesendanger, M. (2006). Eccles' perspective of the forebrain, its role in skilled movement, and the mind-brain problem. *Prog. Neurobiol.* 78, 304–321.

Wills, C. L., F. Cacucci, N. Burgess J. O'Keefe, (2005). Attractor dynamics in the hippocampal representation of the local environment. *Science,* 308 (5723): pp. 873 – 876.

Winnicott, D. W. (1958). *Collected Papers: Through Paediatrics To Psycho-Analysis.* London: Tavistock Publications.

Winnicott, D. W. (1971). *Playing and Reality,* London: Tavistock Publications.

Winslow, J. T., Hastings, N., Carter, C.S., Harbaugh, C.R., Insel, T.R. (1993) A role for central vasopressin in pair bonding in monogamous prairie voles. *Nature.* Oct 7;365(6446):545-8.

Wittgenstein, L. (1967). *Philosophical Investigations,* Oxford: Oxford University Press.

Yoo, H.J., Cho, S.C., Ha, J., Yune, S.K., Kim, S.J., Hwang, J., Chung, A., Sung, Y.H., and Lyoo, I.K. (2004). Attention deficit hyperactivity symptoms and internet addiction, *Psychiatry Clin Neurosci,* 58(5):487-94.

Zanette, D. H. and Mikhailov, A. S. (1998) Condensation in globally coupled populations of chaotic dynamical systems, *Phys. Rev. E* 57(1), 276-281.

Zanette, D. H. and Mikhailov, A. S. (1998b) Mutual synchronization in ensembles of globally coupled neural networks, *Phys. Rev. E* 58(1), 872-875.

Zanette, D. H. and Morelli L. G. (2003) Synchronization Of Coupled Extended Dynamical Systems, *International Journal of Bifurcation and Chaos*, Vol. 13, No. 4.

Zanette, D. H. and Mikhailov, A. S. (2004) Dynamical systems with time-dependent coupling: clustering and critical behaviour, *Physica D* 194 203–218.

Zbilut, J. P., Sirabella, P., Giuliani, A., Manetti, C., Colosimo, A., and Webber, C. L., Jr. (2002). Review of nonlinear analysis of proteins through recurrence quantification. *Cell Biochem.Biophys.,* 36, 67-87.

Zerubavel, E. (1981). *Hidden Rhythms, Schedules And Calendars In Social Life,* Chicago: University of Chicago Press.

Chapter 6

On the Nature and Neural Mechanisms of Mind Force

Walter J. Freeman
Department of Molecular and Cell Biology,
University of California at Berkeley, Berkeley CA, USA

Abstract

A universal characteristic of brains is the existence of background activity. Whether awake or asleep, at rest or in action, brains exhibit continuous high levels of consumption of metabolic energy and the production of waste heat and entropy. The energy is observed in many forms as it acts over distances and creates gradients off electric, magnetic, chemical, and thermal force. The electric forces transmit action and information from the synapse on the dendrite to the trigger zone near the axon hillock. outwardly in excitation and inwardly in inhibition. The chemical forces exerted by the concentration gradients of neurotransmitter molecules released by axon terminals at synapses mediate the transmission of forces between neurons in networks and feedback loops. These forces are steady state and unstructured during rest. During intentional actions the forces become textured both spatially and temporally by self-organization of the background activity. Mind is the structure of the activity of the brain. Mind is then expressed in the intentional behavior that is controlled by the forces exerted by the brain activity on the sensory and motor input/output systems of the brain. The textured neural forces are the Mind Force that is expressed internally in the electrochemical operations inside brains, and consequently in the activities of the body in all fields that are dependent on mind, whether in art, architecture, music, and the interpersonal relationships in psychosocial, economic and political affairs of mankind.

In: Neuroscience and Technology Transform the Educational Ecosystem
Editors: Franco F. Orsucci and Nicoletta Sala
ISBN: 979-8-88697-157-6

1. Introduction

A scientific definition is that Mind Force is the structure of organized brain energy across the cerebral cortex. As in all material systems, energy is force acting over a distance, and power is the rate of dissipation of energy. The neural force of self-organizing activity spreads rapidly over many thousands of cortical columns in the emergence of structure. The brain activity is in multiple types of energy: electrical, magnetic, chemical, thermal, etc. The structures taken by brain energy come in different forms depending on the scales of time and distance that we impose on our observations by the choice of our techniques for recording and measuring brain activity. Our views of the structures also depend on our choice of behavioral correlates.

Mind Force is not restricted to patterns of neuronal firings in cerebral cortex, because those patterns are immediately expressed in the movements of the body. This is because the motor systems of the brain are embedded in the cerebral cortex, and they transmit the cortical dynamic structure to the musculoskeletal system. The relationship is captured in the title of Merleau-Ponty's (1942) most famous book, in which he defined mind as "The Structure of Behavior." Our recognition and understanding of Mind Force inevitably requires us to correlate the arcane and complex patterns of neural activity with organized, intentional behaviors, by means of which each of us expresses our Mind Force. Pari passu each of us experiences the Mind Force of others through our eyes, ears, nose, tongue and body, not through hypothetical channels of empathy, radiation, nonlocality, or other fictional postulates.

The choice of the term "Mind Force" is misleading in one respect, because it may raise in readers the conceptions of telekinesis and the manipulation of objects solely by thinking about them. Such nonsense was popularized by the Israeli magician Uri Geller, who made his living by creating the illusion of bending spoons by his focused attention. His livelihood of entertainment was certainly not fraudulent, but it was not scientific either.

Mind Force was widely adopted in the era of 19th century thermodynamics, which flowered following the demonstration by Herman Helmholtz of the First Law of Thermodynamics: the conservation of energy (Freeman, 1997). Herbert Spencer (1868) wrote that it is "...an unquestionable truth that, at any moment, the existing quantity of liberated nerve-force, which in an inscrutable way produces in us the state we call feeling, must expend itself in some direction — must generate an equivalent manifestation of force somewhere (p. 109)." Charles Darwin (1872) wrote: "This involuntary transmission of nerve force may or may not be accompanied by consciousness.

Why the irritation of nerve-cells should generate or liberate nerve force is not known; but that this is the case seems to be the conclusion arrived at by all the greatest physiologists such as Mueller, Virchow and Bernard, and so on (p. 72).” H. Hughlings Jackson used it in his neurological theories of the involution and devolution of the brain. Sigmund Freud labeled it “Q” when he used it in founding psychoanalysis with his unpublished “Project for a Scientific Psychology.”

The usefulness of equilibrium thermodynamics ended when it became clear that *nerve-energy* is not conserved; brains are open systems. The need for brain theory was met when *nerve-energy* was replaced with *information*, using the same concepts of sources, sinks, channels, channel capacity, and negentropy – new wine in an old bottle (Freeman, 1997). Presently with the growing awareness of the inappropriateness of information theory for describing neural fields of activity, there is increasing recognition of the value of the term Mind Force for describing the neural mechanisms of higher brain functions, but now in the context of nonlinear, far-from-equilibrium thermodynamics (Freeman, 2008).

There are many modes of behaviors in which Mind Force is expressed, ranging from scavenging for food, constructing shelter, seeking companions and mates, pressuring and being pressured by peers, and creating works of art for the pure pleasure of doing so. These correlates are the concerns of psychologists, psychiatrists, anthropologists, sociologists, art critics and historians. The concerns of neuroscientists are directed not to the body but to the brain. We want answers to salient questions. What are the basic forms taken by Mind Force? How is Mind Force generated from metabolic energy? How is the steady-state flow of Mind Force shaped into oscillations in the beta and gamma ranges that are synchronized over wide areas of cerebral cortex? How are the synchronized oscillations parsed into bursts that constitute frames as in a cinema? How are the frames textured in the expression of memories, thoughts, desires, and intentional actions?

Every form of expression of Mind Force requires energy, none more so than the activity of the cerebral cortex. Brains dissipate energy at rates ten times greater than any other organ. Perhaps the most important reason is that cortical neurons sum excitatory and inhibitory potentials that they generate with excitatory and inhibitory synapses. The potentials cancel, but the energy adds as the square of the ionic currents. The discrepancy led Marcus Raichle (2006) to borrow from physics the term “dark energy,” but in brain science the discrepancy is not a mystery.

2. What Are the Basic Forms Taken by Mind Force?

Recordings of electric potentials through microelectrodes reveal a broad range of frequencies of oscillation. Spectral analysis yields power-law distributions of energy. There are two main subdivisions. The frequency range from roughly 1 Hz to 1,000 Hz shows a linear relationship in which the logarithm of power decreases linearly with increasing log frequency. Owing to the linearity the spectrum is designated "1/f." Activity in this range comes mostly from dendritic ionic currents, which are driven by metabolic energy that is released at synapses. This component of brain activity is known as black noise (Schroeder, 1991). It is largely but not totally random. The challenge for neuroscientists is to extract the non-random components from the random noise, because those are signals. Due to the structures they exhibit, they are the manifestations of Mind Force.

The frequency range roughly from 1,000 Hz to 10,000 Hz shows a flat spectrum from the superposition of innumerable action potentials that give a steady roar like the sound of a waterfall. This component is known as white noise. The aim of recording from a microelectrode is to place the electrode close enough to single neurons one at a time to extract a sequence of action potentials called a pulse train. If the pulses in the train come at unpredictable intervals, then the pulse train is random. Then the distribution of pulse intervals is exponential, and the pulse train conforms to a Poisson process. That statistical pattern provides one definition of the rest state of cortex (Freeman, Ahlfors and Menon, 2009). If the intervals between pulses are periodic, or if the pulses occur in short bursts, then the pulses are signals, and they are manifestations of Mind Force.

One of two forms of electric energy expressing Mind Force in cortex is the axonal signal, which is known as the action potential, pulse, spike, and unit. The pulse is the predominant mode of transmission within neurons over distances > 1 mm, which are too great for communication by diffusion. The transmission of signals by pulses is reliable and without attenuation but with a delay. The ionic currents of the pulse flow inside the neuron in one direction, across the membrane where the action is located, and passively outside the neuron in the other direction. That extraneuronal flow establishes a weak local field of potential that is epiphenomenal, but that is the sign of the pulse used by observers to measure neural activity. The other form is the dendritic potential. Its electromotive force is in synapses acting as a battery. The current flows inside the neuron in one direction and outside in the other. The extracellular flow across the resistance of the cortical tissue. Creates an extracellular field of potential that is known as the electroencephalogram (EEG) when recorded from the scalp (Freeman, et al., 2003; Pockett at al., 2009; Ruiz et al., 2010), the electrocorticogram (ECoG) when recorded from the cortical surface (Freeman, 2005), and the local field potential (LFP) when recorded from microelectrodes inserted into the depth of the cortex. These extracellular fields are epiphenomenal; they are much too weak to influence the firing of neurons; moreover the cortex is richly endowed with glial cells, which surround the neurons and offer a low-resistance pathway for the extracellular currents between neurons.

These two forms are closely related statistically. The dendritic forces releasing energy at synapses are triggered by action potentials, in which the strength of ionic current increases with the rate of pulses in trains. The summed dendritic currents at the trigger zones of axons where the ionic currents are converged determine the firing rate of the axon. The relation between dendritic current and axonal firing rate is nonlinear, with an S-shape called sigmoidal. Inhibitory dendritic current drives the axon below threshold. Excitatory dendritic current drives the axon to an upper limit that is imposed by the refractory period. If the axon has just fired, it cannot fire again until it has adequately recovered. These two limits at the axon initial segment impose boundaries on the range of activity for cortex. The range is sufficiently narrow that the conversion of pulse frequencies to dendritic current amplitudes at synapses is confined to a near-linear range. This greatly simplifies modeling of cortical dynamics.

There is a major difference between these two observed manifestations of Mind Force. The pulse is a measure of the activity of a single neuron. It gives the microscopic state variable of neural networks. The dendritic wave results from the sum of ionic currents in the local neighborhood from tens of thousands of neurons. It is a local mean field state variable. Its statistical correlate is the pulse probability wave of the population of neurons, which is an expression of the pulse density of the time-multiplexed signal of the neighborhood. The pulse density and the wave density are macroscopic variables. The microscopic and macroscopic state variables are analogous to the kinetic energy of molecules and the temperature of a gas or liquid. Whereas the pulses in neural networks are treated as binary digits and the synapses are treated as switches and weights, in neural populations the pulses are treated as infinitesimals in ordinary and stochastic differential equations.

3. How Is Mind Force Generated from Metabolic Energy?

The outstanding characteristic of the living brain is its ceaseless background activity, often called *spontaneous*. Indeed the sustained absence of activity is legal evidence of death. In the state of rest the spectra of the field potentials (EEG, ECoG, LFP) conform to 1/f, and the pulse trains conform to a Poisson process, indicating the appearance of Mind Force at rest. The origin of the background activity is demonstrated by an electric shock of the incoming axons to the cortex, which causes a brief increase in activity above the background that decays exponentially to base line. The stronger is the shock, the higher is the excitation, and the more rapid is the exponential decay. A graphic display of the decay rate vs. the response amplitude shows that the decay rate extrapolates to zero as the response goes to threshold (Ch. 8 in Freeman, 2000).

The prolonged exponential decay of the impulse response shows that the excitatory neurons are exciting each other in positive, regenerative feedback. The relation of zero decay to zero response means that the excitatory interaction among the neurons exciting each other is bounded by the refractory periods. The synaptic interconnection density is sufficiently high so that whenever a neuron fires a pulse, it receives back more than on pulse. However, if it has just fired it cannot fire again. The lesson is that the origin of the background activity and of the Mind Force is mutual excitation. The necessary connectivity is available, because 80% of cortical neurons are excitatory, and the overwhelming number of connections each neuron receives are from other cortical neurons. The overall activity is absolutely bounded and therefore stable because of the refractory periods. Inhibition is not necessary.

The background activity is randomized, because each neuron transmits to thousands of other neurons, and it receives input from thousands of others by multiple synaptic loops of one, two, three, etc., synapses over the duration of the exponential decay. The population feedback path can be modeled as a one-dimensional diffusion process, so that the background activity continually and intrinsically undergoes decoherence. That positive feedback among excitatory neurons creates the steady-state background activity from which the signals of structured Mind Force emerge.

First among these departures from randomness is the limitation on firing rates imposed by refractory periods. The power spectral density of the background activity is power-law; log power falls with increasing log frequency in a straight line, $1/f^a$. The slope of the line is not -2 ($a = 2$) as would be expected for randomness (*brown noise*). It is steeper ($2 < a < 4$) (*black noise*, Freeman and Zhai, 2009). The loss of high frequency power over the broad spectrum is due to the refractory periods, which limit the discharge rates of all neurons. Even so, the background activity is not merely a steady-state, zero-frequency excitatory bias; it contains all frequencies in the spectral range of the EEG and the ECoG.

4. How Is the Steady-State Flow of Mind Force Shaped into Oscillations?

Mutual excitation is a form of positive feedback. It supports prolonged firing on brief impulse inputs. The interaction promotes synchrony and co-firing of neurons. Mutual inhibition among inhibitory neurons that inhibit each other is also a form of positive feedback with prolongation of temporal responses. The interaction promotes spatial contrast enhancement (Mach bands), because a neuron that inhibits its neighbor is released from inhibition by that neighbor and tends to fire longer and continue to inhibit its neighbor. Both types of positive feedback generate broad-band oscillations with 1/f temporal spectra that contain all frequencies.

The interaction of excitatory and inhibitory neurons supports narrow-band temporal oscillation that produces local peaks in temporal spectra. The cycle duration in sec (the reciprocal of the frequency in Hz) is determined mainly by the passive membrane time constant of about 5 msec, and partly by the axonal propagation and dendritic cable delays and the synaptic delay, summing to 6.25 msec for each synaptic step.

There are four steps in each cycle: E excites I, I inhibits E, E disexcites I, I disinhibits E, which fires again and initiates the next cycle. Four steps total 25 msec, which is 40 Hz. This is negative feedback.

The two kinds of positive feedback modulate the nominal center frequency over a range of 30 to 80 Hz (Ch. 5 in Freeman, 1975/2004), which is the gamma range. Similar interactions that incorporate longer transmission delays between cortices support oscillations by negative feedback in the beta range (12 to 30 Hz). The beta and gamma together constitute the main activity range of the field potentials.

There is a common misconception that negative feedback is homeostatic and therefore stabilizing, whereas positive feedback is conceived as regenerative and therefore destabilizing.

In practice both kinds of feedback can be stable or unstable. In general the positive feedback that supports the generation of Mind Force is inherently stable and is governed by a point attractor in dynamical models of cortical phase space. The negative feedback that supports the shaping of Mind Force into beta and gamma oscillations is inherently unstable, because the expression of structure in Mind Force is discontinuous. It requires the starting and stopping of oscillations that are imposed or selectively enhanced in the steady state background noise.

5. How Are Synchronized Oscillations Parsed into Bursts Like Cinematic Frames?

Whereas the background activity is broad-band and contains all frequencies, the bursts of oscillations that are initiated by sensory input are narrow-band in the gamma range. The width of the pass band has been estimated from the temporal minimum of the spatial standard deviation, $SD_X(t)$, of the 64 signals that are sampled in each frame. The center frequency jumps unpredictably from each frame to the next, anywhere from 30 to 80 Hz, but the minimal $SD_X(t)$ is relatively constant in the range of 6 to 10 Hz.

The oscillation superimposed on the background acts like a band pass filter. Stephen Rice (1950) has shown that the addition of such narrow band oscillation to random activity results in *beats* that cause waxing and waning of the amplitude of the oscillation.

The distribution of the intervals between beats was predicted by Rice to depend solely on the width of the pass band, independently of the center frequency. Measurement of the modal intervals showed that they corresponded to the wavelengths of oscillations in the theta range (Freeman, 2009).

The high segments of the beats appeared as bursts in the ECoG. The low segments of beats were found to contain one or more extremely low values, on the order of a decrease by 10^{-4} to 10^{-6} below the mean power of the signals which were named n*ull spikes* (Freeman, 2009).

During this null spike the EGoG signal in the pass band of the bursts showed an abrupt phase resetting, indicating that the null spike led to an indeterminacy of the phase, and the conditions necessary for a phase transition.

It was postulated that the decrease in interaction among the cortical neurons during beats created an opportunity for the cortex to terminate an existing spatial pattern and initiate a new pattern, which was selected from memory by the action of a sensory stimulus impacting the cortex.

The null spikes preferentially recurred in the theta frequency range, as predicted by our calculations using the statistical distributions discovered and developed by Rice (1950).

6. How Are Frames Textured in the Expression of Memories and Actions?

Sensory information is expressed in the firing of action potentials by single neurons and local networks of neurons. Mind Force is guided by information that it takes from the action potentials, but the currency of Mind Force is knowledge that is constructed from information. This process begins in the sensory cortices, which receive action potentials either directly from sensory receptor in olfaction or by relays through pre-processing networks in all other sensory systems. Sensory receptors are vastly redundant with substantial convergence from receptor arrays to cortices. The task of generalization over equivalent receptors is carried out by the formation under reinforcement learning of Hebbian nerve cell assemblies, one for each conditioned stimulus that a subject can discriminate. Synapses between pairs of co-excited excitatory neurons are strengthened in associative learning and weakened in habituation. Over multiple trials the cortex forms a correlation map, in which activation of any subset subsequently excites the entire cell assembly in the stereotypic expression of the category of the stimulus, regardless of which among equivalent receptors were activated. When the assembly is activated by a stimulus, the oscillation in the frame shows a spatial pattern of amplitude modulation (AM) (Barrie, Freeman and Lenhart, 1996; Freeman, 2005). The AM pattern is never twice identical but it is sufficiently distinctive to allow classification of frames in groups far above chance levels. From this it is concluded that the AM pattern is the element in the code used by Mind Force to disseminate its perceptual knowledge that it constructed from sensory information.

This formation of an agency for generalization takes place very quickly, within a few trials. In the next 24 hours consolidation takes place in which the cell assembly is embedded in a much larger synaptic matrix that incorporates other parts of the brain, such as the limbic system. The embedding enriches the contextual associations of the cortical response to a stimulus, so that the knowledge that is transmitted is not just the category of the stimulus but its significance for the subject and what the subject should do with the sensory information.

Conclusion

The sensory receptor arrays express sensory information in trains of action potentials and transmit the pulses by axon arrays that are topographically organized. The dynamics of sensory cortex uses the microscopic information that is expressed in the topographically organized sensory discharges to construct knowledge about the stimuli and expresses it in spatial patterns of macroscopic neural mass action. The mass action patterns cannot be observed with existing techniques for single neuron recording, because the populations are too large for current sampling techniques. They can be observed and measured by recording the EEG and ECoG with arrays of electrodes, and the metabolic costs can be assayed with fMRI (Freeman, Ahlfors and Menon, 2009). Each channel receives contributions from 10^4 to 10^5 cortical neurons, so each signal qualifies as a macroscopic variable. The spatial patterns of neural mass action are scale-free, with self-similarity over patterns sizes ranging from a few sq. mm. to the entire surface of the scalp. The implication is that local and global macroscopic patterns are readily combined by the embedding of multiple patterns at different carrier frequencies, owing to the self-similarity. How this interaction may take place is unknown, and is a prime target for research.

References

Barrie J M, Freeman W J, Lenhart M (1996). Modulation by discriminative training of spatial patterns of gamma EEG amplitude and phase in neocortex of rabbits. *J. Neurophysiology* 76: 520-539.

Darwin C (1872). *The Expression of Emotions in Man and Animals*. London: Murray.

Freeman W J (1975). *Mass Action in the Nervous System*. New York: Academic Press. © 2004 http://sulcus.berkeley.edu/MANSWWW/MANSWWW.html.

Freeman W J (1997). Three centuries of category errors in studies of the neural basis of consciousness and intentionality. *Neural Networks* 10: 1175-1183.

Freeman W J (2000). *Neurodynamics: An Exploration of Mesoscopic Brain Dynamics*. London: Springer.

Freeman W J (2005). Origin, structure, and role of background EEG activity. Part 3. Neural frame classification. *Clin. Neurophysiol.* 116 (5): 1118-1129. http://repositories.cdlib.org/postprints/2134/

Freeman W J [2008]. A pseudo-equilibrium thermodynamic model of information processing in nonlinear brain dynamics. *Neural Networks* 21: 257-265. http://repositories.cdlib.org/postprints/2781.

Freeman W J (2009). Deep analysis of perception through dynamic structures that emerge in cortical activity from self-regulated noise. *Cognitive Neurodynamics* 3(1): 105-116. http://www.springerlink.com/content/v375t5l4t065m48q/

Freeman, W J, Burke, B C and Holmes, M D [2003]. Aperiodic phase re-setting in scalp EEG of beta-gamma oscillations by state transitions at alpha-theta rates. *Human Brain Mapping* 19(4):248-272. http://repositories.cdlib.org/postprints/3347.

Freeman W J, Kozma R (2010). Freeman's mass action. *Scholarpedia*, 5(1): http://www.scholarpedia.org/article/Freeman%27s_mass_action http://www.springer .com/math/numbers/book/978-3-540-69394-9.

Freeman W J, Zhai J (2009). Simulated power spectral density (PSD) of background electrocorticogram (ECoG). *Cognitive Neurodynamics* 3(1): 97-103. http://repositories.cdlib.org/postprints/3374.

Kozma R, Huntsberger T, Aghazarian H, Tunstel E, Ilin R, Freeman W J [2008]. Implementing intentional robotics principles using SSR2K platform. *Advanced Robotics* 22(12): 1309-1327.

Merleau-Ponty M (1942/1963). *The Structure of Behavior* (Fischer AL, Trans.). Boston: Beacon Press.

Pockett S, Bold G E J, Freeman W J (2009). EEG synchrony during a perceptual-cognitive task: Widespread phase synchrony at all frequencies. *Clin. Neurophysiol.* 120: 695-708. doi:10.1016/j.clinph.2008.12.044.

Raichle M E (2006). The brain's dark energy. *Science* 314: 1249-1250.

Rice S O (1950). *Mathematical Analysis of Random Noise* - and Appendixes – Technical Publications Monograph B-1589. New York: Bell Telephone Labs Inc.

Ruiz Y, Pockett S, Freeman W J, Gonzales E, Li Guang (2010). A method to study global spatial patterns related to sensory perception in scalp EEG. *J. Neuroscience Methods* 191: 110-118.

Schroeder M (1991). *Fractals, Chaos, Power Laws*. Minutes from an Infinite Paradise. San Francisco: WH Freeman.

Spencer H (1868). *Essays: Scientific, Political, and Speculative*. London: Williams.

Chapter 7

An Inquiry/Review into the Generalized Spectrum of Dimensions, D_q, and Its Relevance to Research*

Frederick David Abraham†
Blueberry Brain Institute, Waterbury, Vermont, USA

Abstract

The generalized spectrum of dimensions of time series provides additional measures of a signal that single dimensional measures fail to offer: (1) when a single dimension is chosen it may not discriminate between experimental conditions when other choices might have succeeded. Running the spectrum provides a search of all possible dimensional measures. (2) parameters of the spectrum provide additional features such as asymptotes, inflections, etc. that may also reveal the effects of different experimental conditions. The use of multiple methods of measurement and the use of a comprehensive approach to experimental design and analysis is urged. Thus we examine an application of the generalized dimensions and graphic EEG presentation (Kulish, Sourin, & Sourina, 2006), and a comprehensive program of data analysis (Sprott, 2003).

---

* This article was originally published in Chaos and Complexity Letters, volume 4 number 2 (2010).
† Corresponding Author's Email: abraham@pshift.com.

In: Neuroscience and Technology Transform the Educational Ecosystem
Editors: Franco F. Orsucci and Nicoletta Sala
ISBN: 979-8-88697-157-6

1. Introduction

Nonlinear measures of the dimensionality, D_q, of time series have usually used methods that yield a single dimension, such as the capacity dimension, q = 0), the information dimension, (q = 1), and the correlation dimension, (q = 2), to name the most familiar. D_2, developed by Grassberger & Procaccia (1983), is the most tractable and meaningful of these for experimental data. But D_q can be generalized for q as a continuous variable over a large range as a generalized spectrum of dimensions, also known as multifractals (Grassberger, 1983; Hentschel & Procaccia, 1983; Paladin & Vulpiani, 1987; Rényi, 1970) and well presented in (Abarbanel, 1996; Kantz & Schreiber, 1997; Ott, Sauer, & Yorke, 1994; Sprott, 2003). Despite the potential for improved information about the differences in experimental data that the D_q offers there are few applications that have been made to real data, but there are a few on the dynamics of heartbeat (Amaral et al., 2001), EEG (Kulish, Sourin, & Sourina, 2006), and tropical rainforest (Solé & Manrubia, 1995). My purpose here is not to develop further the methodology, but (a) to try to emphasize its potential usefulness in order to get more researchers to explore that potential, and (b) to review overall data-analytic strategies in which this method would be imbedded. The strategy is mainly that of Sprott (2003) whose comprehensive program is outstanding but, unfortunately, seldom used.

I start with an examination of the Kulish et al., paper on EEG and language. They state their goal as "developing new methods of processing data recorded by well-established techniques [that] may prove useful while deeper penetrating into the mystery of human consciousness." Since the brain is non-linear and FFT power spectral analyses are linear, non-linear measures should prove useful. Their use of the D_q is valuable in that regard. I also include a presentation of their graphic methods of evaluating EEG because multiple methods of evaluating signal differences complement each other. I comment on ways of increasing the cross-relevance of their dimensional and graphic methods in my 'wish list,' a discussion of research design and analysis strategies.

Note that it is reasonable to consider that the linear spectra of frequency decomposition of time signals is indeed useful, but that multiple analytic methods might supplement with additional information that can be extracted from the signal(s) including nonlinear and graphic measures. For example, in R. Abraham & C. Shaw (*Dynamics: The Geometry of Behavior*), they have a figure comparing the representations of various attractors with three images each: the portrait, the time series, and the frequency spectrum (Part 2,

Figure 4.5.7; repeated in Abraham, Abraham, & Shaw, Figure II-49. These books also show the relationship to characteristic exponents (Liapunov exponents), but not to fractal dimension, the subject of this paper). As Abarbanel (1996, p. 69) puts it, "Since chaotic motion produces continuous broadband Fourier spectra, we clearly have to replace narrowband Fourier signatures with other characteristics of the system for purposes of identification and classification." Then he mentions fractal dimensions and Lyapunov exponents as the two main candidates as classifiers.

2. Mathematical Analysis

Kulish et al., begin with the Rényi entropy measure, which seemed curious at first since it does not use sequential properties of the data, but rather is the probability distribution function of the time signal (i.e., the EEG voltages). Buat from it they developed the generalized fractal dimension, D_q, the convolution over the probability distributions of order q summed over the bins of the EEG voltages and the size of the hypersphere, δV (which is equivalent to r or ε of the usual formulations of D since there is a measured dimension, voltage, associated with r). This is their equation 6 (Sprott, §13.2.2, eqn. 13.14, p. 338; Kant & Schrieber, §11.3.1 eqn. 11.12, p. 187; Ott, Sauer, Yorke, §2.2, eqn. 2.2, p. 15; Abarbanel, §5.2, eqn. 5.12, p. 73, Renyi, 1970; Grassberger, 1983; Hentschel & Procaccia, 1983; Paladin & Vulpiani, 1987). The resulting D_q as a function of q, is sometimes called the fractal spectrum, also, the generalized Renyi entropy, generalized fractal dimensions, generalized dimensions, the spectrum of fractional dimensions, multifractal spectrum of dimensions, and multifractal.

Further, the generalized fractal dimensions of a given time series with a known probability distribution are defined by the equation

$$D_q = \lim_{\delta V \to 0} \frac{1}{q-1} \frac{\log \sum_{i=1}^{N} p_i^q}{\log \delta V},$$

Of the four books I have mentioned, any one of them presents a more than adequate presentation of the mathematics involved, but each has strengths that warrant owning all of these books. Abarbanel's (1996) is excellent for data visualization, especially on explaining the box counting method with figures for the Hénon attractor (reproduced in Abraham, 1997). Kantz & Scheiber's

(1997) is especially good in pointing out (a) the pitfalls when applying the techniques (§6.4), (b) when automated algorithmic methods work well, and (c) when the art of looking at the graphics of intermediate steps is needed in an analysis. They also caution about the of loss of information in trying to characterize a dynamic by reduction to single numbers - e.g., p. 38 on visual inspection of data; p. 72 on independence from measurement and analysis parameters. They are also good on stressing the use of multiple approaches to data analyses. They have an appendix containing some of their numerical routines in both Fortran and C. Ott et al., (1994) have a unique organization by with general explanatory chapters each of which is followed by many reprints of classic original papers, a must-have reference work from that perspective. Sprott (2003) is excellent for (a) clear explanations, (b) completeness, (c) appendices including a huge list with summaries of known attractors, (d) historical vignettes on many the authors in the history of dynamics, and (e) a web site that helps with exercises and which keeps the book constantly updated.

3. Experimental Technique and Signal Processing

I was surprised to see EEG of 10-15 mV p/p; sure beats the days when I did EEG from indwelling electrodes (theirs was scalp), which might explain why they could be so casual with respect to shielding and isolation of the subjects, and with respect to grounding issues (not enough information but I assume they had no problem with ground loops). Mine (indwelling, cat) were more in the range reported by Babloyantz (1988/1990, see Figure 2 showing typical ranges of EEG voltages) At any rate, their signals looked pretty clean. I was curious about their putting cotton balls behind the ears. Could that have been for EOG rather than ECG? A misprint? Statistical processing and "the significance test was performed." Which tests and on what?

Their behavioral task consisted of asking the subject a question to which they had to respond 'yes' or 'no.' Then they performed the D_q on the EEG to each of these responses. The precise timing of the analysis period and the response was not given. Presumably, these EEG samples were taken during the utterance, although the 5 sec EEG sample is considerably longer than the utterance of the answer would take.

4. Fractal Spectra of EEGs

They state that the Fourier transform does not yield information about amplitude, but it does provide amplitude information in a relative sense at least (power per frequency band; when the signal is in arbitrary units), and can be true in the absolute sense of the distribution of $V^2/\delta f$ as a function of f if calibrations are made which reveal the transfer function of the measuring system (*sans* electrode/brain interface in our work (Abraham, F. D. Brown, D., & Gardiner, M. (1968). Hard to believe it had never been done before. We did it with a train of rectangular pulses whose convolution yielded the whole spectrum with a single signal.) While they accuse the Fourier of also not yielding fractionality information, it is just as true that while the fractal dimension is sensitive to frequency information, it does not yield any frequency information directly. Is it hard to believe that if the D_q discriminated between the responses, the Fourier would also not yield a difference if performed with appropriate parametric choices? These are minor points and not very consequential considering the important methods that they are developing.

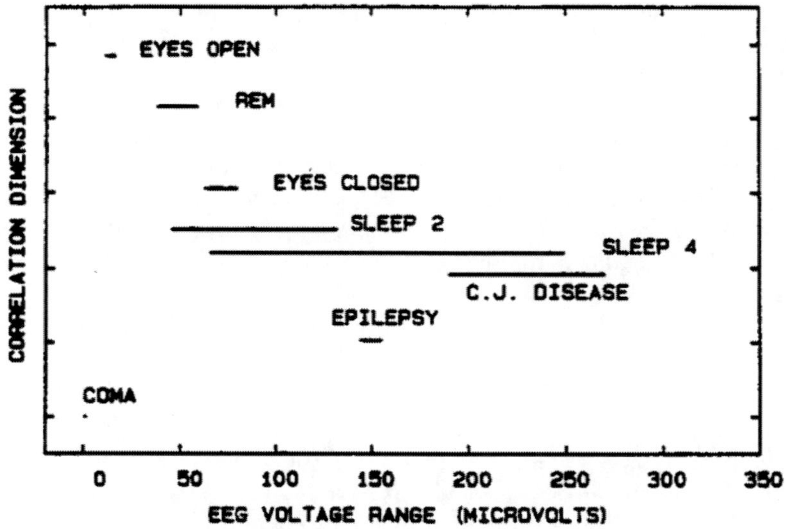

Figure 1. Dimension-amplitude plot. The variations of EEG voltage observed at the optimal sampling frequencies (see text) and in successive stretches of 1 s are represented for each type of EEG behavior. The synchronization between neurons which occur in pathologies is reflected by high amplitudes and low dimensions.

While the EEG voltages may have been large compared to EEGs reported earlier, the opposite is true for the fractal dimensions. After Grassberger & Procaccia first reported their algorithms for measuring D_2 in 1983, there were a spate of articles reporting D_2 and attractor reconstructions for EEG, mostly with D_2s of 4-6 compared to the <2 values reported in Kulish (Başar & bullock, 1989; Başar, 1990, see Table 2, Introduction) 2. Why might this be? One can only speculate, since there were not many details of the analysis procedures given. But perhaps we can get a clue from Kantz & Scheriber (1997), §6.3, where they point out that calculating the correlation sum and dimension involve attractor reconstruction, which involves the delay imbedding procedure (where calculating the delay τ is critical); "A value which "yields a convincing phase portrait should do for the correlation sum as well." Also, results should be "invariant under reasonable changes to the embedding procedure" (p. 73).

> "Once the embedding vectors are reconstructed, the estimation of dimension is done in two steps," determining the correlation sum, $C(m,\varepsilon)$, where m is the embedding dimension, ε (= r of others), the radius of the covering hypersphere) and then "inspect $C(m, \varepsilon)$ for signatures of self-similarity. If these signatures are convincing enough, we can compute a value for the dimension. Both steps require some care in order to avoid wrong or misleading results" (p. 73).
>
> "The straightforward estimator, Eqn. (6.1), turns out to be biased toward too small dimensions when the pairs entering the sum are not statistically independent. For time series data with nonzero autocorrelations, independence cannot be assumed. ... The most important temporal correlations are caused by the fact that data close in time are also close in space" [For the EEG in Kulish et al., the state space is based on voltage]. "It is more than likely that the majority of dimension estimates published for field measurements are seriously too low because they mistake temporal coherence for geometrical structure." (Kantz & Schreiber, p. 73; demonstrated by Theiler, 1986).

The solution involves decimating the time series to eliminate the correlations. Kantz & Schreiber's next section, 6.4, shows how $C(\varepsilon)$ as a function of ε and $d(\varepsilon)$ as a function of ε with parameter m is examined for linear portions (those signatures of self-similarity). The finite nature of the attractor and differing densities of points at different portions of the attractor affect the statistical reliability.

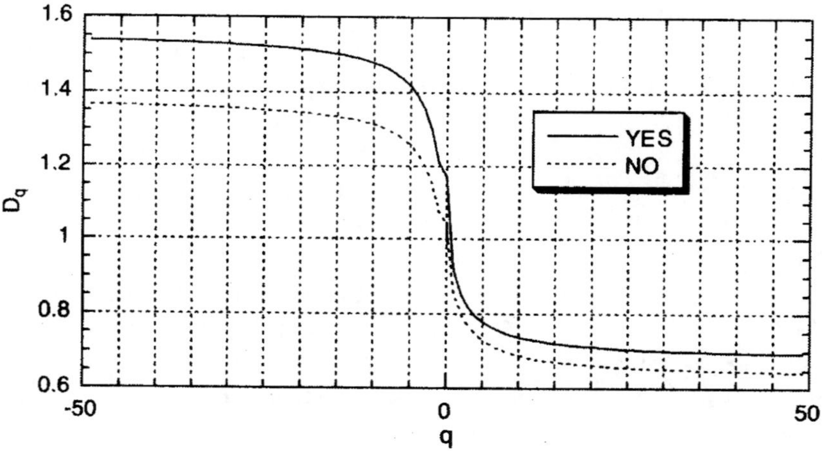

Figure 2. The sample averaged fractal spectra of EEGs.

Sprott summarizes some 11 steps or procedures for the analysis of time series data (Sprott, §13.8; summarized here in §6 below). Many of these procedures are not mentioned or utilized or are incompletely described in the Kulish paper, so no estimate can be made if their procedures satisfy these precautions. Nonetheless, the use of the apectrum of generalized dimensions, D_q, is an extremely important contribution.

One might remember that in reconstruction work, a usual criterion for selecting a lag, τ, is to use the delay required for the autocorrelation to decay from 1 to 0.

Their main results for one subject are in their Figure 3, and averaged over all subjects, substantially identical, are in their Figure 4. They certainly are well behaved. The curves for "yes" answers are higher than for "no" answers, as is D_0 (Hausdorff-Besicovitch version). In addition, the range of D's from $D_{-\infty}$ to $D_{+\infty}$ was also greater for "yes" than "no" answers. Following the latter result, they state, "Hence, the 'YES' spectra are *on the average* more fractal than the 'NO' spectra. This implies that the brain is *on the average* more active while answering 'YES' question. In addition, it is evident from Figure 4 that *on the average*, more unexpected values are present in the 'YES' signal, whereas the 'NO' signal is *on the average more* predictable and uniform."

The conclusion that the spectra are greater for the "yes" answers certainly seems safe, even without error boundaries for the curves. The conclusion that the brain is more active is not necessarily wrong, but requires some conjecturing to have any meaning. It is consistent with the typical results, e.g., the Figure 1 above (taken from Babloyantz (1989/1990) which shows D_2 as a function of voltage for disease (epilepsy, Creutzfeld-Jakob), sleep (stages 2, 4, and REM), and eyes closed and open, with D_2s increasing from about 2 to 10 (as voltage ranges decrease). A clue to interpreting such a result is given by Babloyantz: "The synchronization between neurons which occur in pathologies is reflected by high amplitudes and low dimensions." (see caption of her figure). That is, it is not necessarily more or less activity, but the coherence of neuronal activity that is being broken down into subpopulations of neurons and involved in more information processing tasks occurring at any time (also, see Abraham, 1997; Abraham et al., 1973 on coherence and brain transactions). Why would "yes" involve such an increase in information processing in the brain. While it is impossible to tell from this experiment, or to conjecture with any confidence (i.e., regarding the involvement of greater emotion, less security, more information to evaluate cognitively), it would be of value to use signal-detection theoretical methodology and interrogation of the research participants to try to understand emotional and cognitive strategies.

What do we make of the fact that the range of D_q is greater for "yes" than "no"? Probably not much. The increase was due to the negative end of the spectra (where $q < 0$) which is more sensitive to the less dense portions of the attractor, which is where the more extreme voltages are. Mutlifractals are designed to overcome problems of committing to a particular D due to the variability in the density (probability of occupancy) of the attractor. Sprott (2003, p. 338): "The limit [of D_q as] q approaches $+\infty$ gives the local dimension in the most densely populated region of the attractor, and the limit q approaches $-\infty$ gives the local dimension in the least densely populated region. The former can be calculated more accurately than the latter because there are usually many more points in the denser region (which is how it got to be dense!)."

The "yes" signal has more unexpected values; the "no" more predictable. Do we need D_q to tell us that? Not only is it obvious from the time signal (EEG), but wouldn't a simple frequency (probability) distribution and/or its statistical moments tell us the same? Doesn't this result tell us as much about D than D does about predictability? Of course the big question is: does signal predictability reflect cognitive predictability? This is an interesting question that should be amenable to further experimentation.

Kulish et al., comment that the information dimension, D_1, higher for "yes" than "no," is unexpected since they should have "equal informational content." However it is not necessarily the case that the cognitive and emotional requirements (nor the brain processes required) for the two answers should be the same, and indeed, the fact that the whole spectrum (not just D_1), is different for the two answers would seem to indicate that to be the case. But with the respect to the EEG signal, D_1, which equals the limit of the Shannon entropy [Sprott: "the amount of information required to specify the state of the system"] divided by log δV as δV approaches 0, which as Sprott observes, "describes how fast the information needed to specify a point on the attractor increases as r [δV in this paper] decreases." (Sprott, 203, p. 339).

Kulish et al., make a further conjecture that "this result [unequal D_1s] can be viewed as an indirect proof of the fact that the operation of the brain is fuzzy, that is there is an overlap between the set in question ("YES") and its complement ("NO")." Very indirect!! Fuzzy?! What can this mean? While yes and no may be complementary as far as the language goes, the expectation that completely different brain processes might support them is an unlikely hypothesis. Suppose the brain was divided into two sets of neurons that only talked to neurons in their own set. Might we not have achieved the same result? And why, as they claim, should the D_1s add up to 2 bits as they claim? [$D_{1,yes}$ = 0.921 bits; $D_{1,no}$ = 0.853 bits; Σ = 1.774 bits, whereas, if independent the sum should be 2 bits according to Kulish et al., I am a bit confused as I didn't think the limits defining D, even the information dimension D_1 had units or dimension of their own, so this argument escapes me; but I am on unsure ground on this]. Babloyantz "eyes closed" and eyes open" conditions each had D_2s (which must be very close to D_1 as the D_q curves all have the same shape, and adjacent D_qs are very similar) >2. There likely is an overlap in the processing of information in making the binary decision, but it is hard for me to see how it follows from the non-additivity of D_1s of the EEGs for the two responses. In a final observation about the fractal results, Kulish et al., point out that the D_q curves are nearly identical to that for the logistic equation (but they don't specify the parameter of the logistic).

It may be relevant that Sprott shows nearly identical curves for the logistic equation (he specifies the logistic equation's constant for different multifractals and approximates the logistic with an asymmetrical Cantor set, (§13.4.2, Figure 13.11, pp. 342-243) and for a pair of asymmetric Cantor sets (§13.3.1, Figure 13.8, pp. 340-341). [One might note, *a la* the Kulish argument, that these curves do share the same brain, that is the same equation except for control parameters, with the sum of D_1s in the neighborhood of 1].

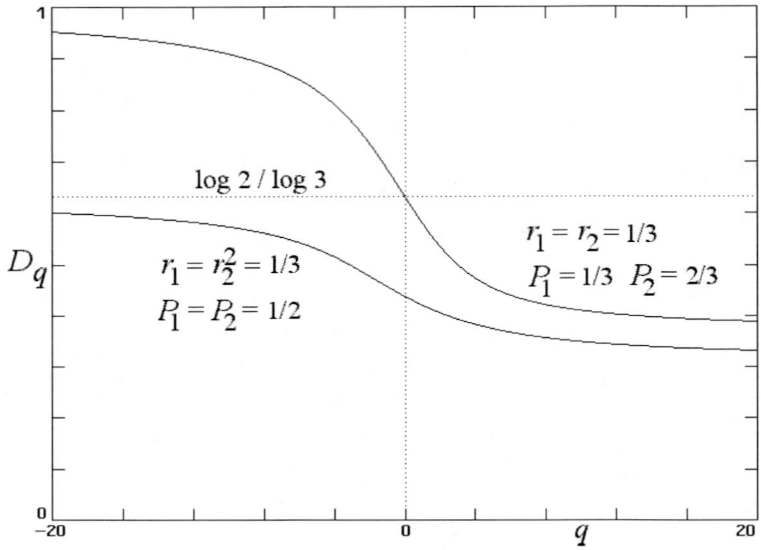

Figure 3. D_q for two different asymmetric Cantor sets. (Thanks to Sprott for sending an electronic copy of figure 13.8, from Sprott, 2003, p. 341).

The fact that two identical deterministic difference equations deferring only in the choice of their parameters yield similar curves whose difference can be specified with but a few parameters (amplitude and range of D_q, D_0, slope of the tangent at the inflection point at D_0) does not imply that two real-world processes, such as the cognitive ability to answer 'yes' or 'no' to questions, are generated by either similar or different processes. Nor does it tell you whether even the processes are deterministic or stochastic (where the difference equations for the latter would have to have a probabilistic component). It does mean that the dimensional magnitude of one is greater than the other. If deterministic equations represent similar processes, in what way are they fuzzy other than that they shared some components of a process but not others? Because an attractor is chaotic or possesses fractal dimension and can be characterized with Shannon entropy neither makes nor disproves the probabilistic case. For those who wish to involve stochastic resonance, specific theories would have to built on the brain/cognitive processes involved in which noise contributes to hill climbing from the basin of one attractor into that of another, and I suspect such attempts would likely to be rather simplifications or the several cognitive/emotional processes involved.

5. Visualization

This is a really exciting methodology, and its potential use in psychophysical and psychological research and medical diagnosis and therapy is vast. I am not current on what other similar methodologies might be around, but this one looks sophisticated to me.

In brief, the magnitude of EEG is evaluated at each point on the skull, which can be tracked in real time with a visualization by means of 'blobbies,' partial spherical forms on a mannequin head, by means of a graphics computer technology by an award winning distinguished team of biomedical engineers.

The "blobby" is defined by their equation 12, p. 298:

Equation 2

$$f(x, y, z, t) = \sum_{i}^{24} a_i e^{-r_i \cdot b_i(t)} - g \geqslant 0,$$

$$r_i = \sqrt{(x - x_i)^2 + (y - y_i)^2 + (z - z_i)^2},$$

"where *a* is a scale factor, *b* is an exponent scale factor and *g* is a threshold value."

The index *i* is over the EEG channels. *x,y,z* were coordinates in a 3D Cartesian space around each electrode position, and I presume when unindexed, some sort of average. The distance of the electrode to the reference position being r_i. The voltages enter via *b*, and are thus the factor that affects the size of the blobby. More than one blobby can be shown at a time to compare different aspects of an experiment and different loci of activity and their magnitude. The threshold g requires a level of EEG activity before a blobby is visualized for any given electrode location. A blobby is calculated for a given time position, but this can be advanced for real time movies or snapshots for particular time windows, advancing through the 5 sec of the response window.

Here is an example of the first and second .77 sec epochs during an experiment, showing blobbies superimposed on the head for 'yes' and 'no' responses, the color difference surviving as shades of gray here and in the article. It nicely shows the reduced area of cortical activation (it became more so over the ensuing 6 epochs) (Notice the original 256 Hz digitization rates are decimated in half). Interactive computer windows and palettes allow real time changing of both viewing and computational parameters. Boolian operations allow additional experimental evaluations.

They conclude that EEG activity is greater for ‘yes’ responses, but that “no” responses require less mental activity and is more stressful assumed from its lesser cortical involvement but greater persistence in the visual cortex. It is interesting to compare this computerized effort to an early attempt to make such a visualization by Walter and Shipton (1951).

Despite the sophistication of the visualization methods, I think there are other measurements in addition to EEG amplitude including power spectra and co-spectra, and especially EEG coherence measures, and most especially, some of the parameters of the generalized fractal spectra that could be fed into the visualization procedures that might help with more subtle cognitive interpretations. Additionally, I would love to see more complete results for the experiment, and think that any conclusions based on such a brief methodological report would be very exciting when used in a more extensive and rigorous experimental context.

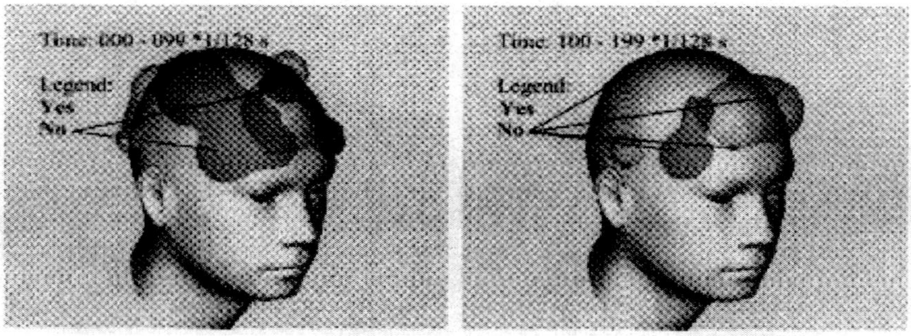

Figure 4. Visualization of EEG activity. From their Figure 6, p. 300.

6. My Wish List

a. When unusual statistical and geometrical representations are used, whether D_q or blobbies, for which the probability distribution functions and their higher moments (variance, skewness, kurtosis) may not be estimated, it is often helpful to evaluate their reliability and significance with Monte Carlo methods. They would constitute a welcome addition to the present study. (Abraham et al., 1973; Abraham, 1997).

b. It is nice to have calibration of EEG signals and their derivative measures demonstrated (Abraham, Brown, & Gardiner, 1968).
c. Utilizing as many of Sprott's 11 steps or procedures for the analysis of time series data as possible (quoted or précis from Sprott, 2003 §13,8, pp. 348-349:

- Make sure the data are free of errors.
- Test for stationarity.
- Explore a variety of plotting the data.
- Determine the correlation time or minimum of the autocorrelation or mutual information to optimize the sampling rate.
- Check the autocorrelation function or fourier spectra for periodicities.
- Make a time-space plot to be sure there are enough data.
- Use false nearest neighbor or saturation to establish the embedding dimension in the determination of D_2.
- If the embedding dimension is low, determine D_2.
- If there is a low dimensional attractor, compute Lyapunov exponents, entropy, and growth rate of unpredictability. If high, remove noise.
- If there is chaos, use surrogate methods for the above tests.
- If there is low dimensional chaos, construct equations and make short-term predictions. If high dimensional chaos (more common), "some predictability [maybe] is possible, and whose power spectrum and probability distribution allow comparison with theoretical models."

d. Considering the subtlety, multiplicity, and complexity of transactions within the brain, and the largely unknown nature of them for the subtleties of cognitive processes, it is not surprising that the best of our analytic techniques are frustratingly inadequate at revealing those subtleties. I am particularly thinking of the relationships which may be taking place between different areas of cortical (and subcortical when indwelling electrodes permit), so when blobbies indicated more than one active area, it could prove of interest to see if the EEG in those areas would show some covariance/coherence (Abraham, 1997; Abraham et al., 1973 for power spectra, but could be done with with

$b_{i,j}$ here). And in fact, all pair-wise sets of electrode results could be funneled into a discriminant or other canonical correlational analysis. And especially, these analyses could be fed into another round of blobby movies.

e. When this paper segued to the visualization I thought they were going to visualize D_q, or at least D_0, D_1, or D_2, or defining parameters of Dq, so I put that on my wish list also. If you put all these together, blobbies for D, voltage, and paired covariance of voltage, along with Monte Carlo and surrogate methods, and the rest of Sprott's steps, then the methods so cleverly developed here would more definitely realize their potential.

f. And finally, some refinement of reporting of experimental procedures, such as the temporal indication of stimuli and response with the EEG recording would prove a benefit. Someone taking advantage of all of these would then be on the threshold of the evolution of an exciting experimental program.

Conclusion

This work described the generalized spectrum of dimensions of time series which provide additional measures of a signal that single dimensional. The use of multiple methods of measurement and the use of a comprehensive approach to experimental design and analysis is urged.

The authors are to be congratulated and thanked for developing these tools for the rest of us to use. I am certainly appreciative of the opportunity to learn as much as possible from this exercise of trying to understand their work, despite my own limitations. I submit it here in hopes that others will become interested in this work and that of the other authors cited.

References

Abarbanel, H. D. I. (1996). *Analysis of observed chaotic data*. New York: Springer-Verlag.

Abraham, F. D. (1997). Nonlinear coherence in multivariate research: Invariants and the reconstruction of attractors. *Nonlinear Dynamics, Psychology & Life Science,* 1, 7-34.

Abraham, F. D. Brown, D., & Gardiner, M. (1968). Calibration of EEG power spectra. *Communications in Behavioral Biology,* 1, 31-36.

Abraham, F. D. Brown, D., & Gardiner, M. (1968). Calibration of EEG power spectra. *Communications in Behavioral Biology,* 1, 31-36.

Abraham, F. D. Bryant, H., Mettler, M., Bergerson, W., Moore, F., Maderdrut, J., Gardiner, M., Walter, D., & Jennrich, R (1973). Spectrum and discriminant analyses reveal remote rather than local sources for hypothalamic EEG: Could waves affect unit activity? *Brain Research,* 49, 349-366.

Abraham, F. D. Bryant, H., Mettler, M., Bergerson, W., Moore, F., Maderdrut, J., Gardiner, M., Walter, D., & Jennrich, R (1973). Spectrum and discriminant analyses reveal remote rather than local sources for hypothalamic EEG: Could waves affect unit activity? *Brain Research,* 49, 349-366.

Abraham, F. D., Abraham, & Shaw, C. D. (1990). *A visual introduction to dynamical systems theory in psychology*. Santa Cruz: Aerial.

Abraham, R. H., & Shaw, C. D. (1988). *Dynamics: The Geometry of Behavior,* Part 2. Santa Cruz: Aerial.

Amaral, L. A. N., Ivanov, P. C., Aoyagi, N., Hidaka, I., Tomono, S., Goldgerger, A. L., Stanley, H. E., & Yamamoto, Y. (2001). Behavioral-independent features of complex heartbeat dynamics. *Physical Review Letters*, 86, 6026-6029.

Babloyantz, A. (1989/1990). Estimation of correlation dimensions from single and multichannel recordings, (in E. Başar & T. H. Bullock, (Eds.), 1989, *Brain dynamaics,* vol 2, pp. 122-130; also reprinted in E. Başar (Ed.), 1990, *Chaos in brain function.*) Berlin, Heidelberg: Springer-Verlag.

Başar, E. (Ed.), 1990, *Chaos in brain function*. Berlin, Heidelberg: Springer-Verlag.

Başar, E., & Bullock, T. H. (Eds.), (1989). *Brain dynamaics,* vol 2.

Grassberger, P. (1983). Generalized dimensions of strange attractors. *Physics Letters A*, 97, 227-230.

Grassberger, P., & Procaccia, I. (1983). Measuring the strangeness of strange attractors. *Phsica D*, 9, 189-208.

Hentschel, H. G. E., & Procaccia, I. (1983). The infinite number of generalized dimensions of fractals and strange attractors. *Physica D*, 8, 435-844.

Kantz, H., & Schreiber, T. (1997). *Nonlinear time series analysis*. Cambridge: Cambridge.

Kulish V., Sourin, A. Sourina, O. (2006). *Computers in Biology and Medicine*, 36, 291-302.

Ott, E., Sauer, T., & Yorke, J. A. (1994). *Coping with chaos: Analysis of chaotic data and the exploitation of chaotic systems*. New York: Wiley.

Paladin, G., & Vulpiani, A. (1987). Anomalous scaling laws in multifractal objects. *Physics Reports*, Alous scaling laws in multifractal objects. *Physics Reports,* 156, 147-225, 147-225.

Renyi, A. (1970). *Probability theory*. Amsterdam: North-Holland.

Solé, R. V., & Manrubia, S. C. (1995). Self-similarity in rain forests: Evidence for a critical state. *Physical Review E*, 51, 6250-6253.

Sprott, J. C. (2003). *Chaos and time-series analysis*. Oxford: Oxford.

Theiler, J. (1986). Spurious dimension from correlation algorithms applied to limited time series data. *Physical Review A*, 34, 2427-2432.

Walter, W. G., & Shipton, H. W. (1951), A new toposcopic display system. *EEG Clin. Neurophsiol.,* 3, 281-292.

Chapter 8

Gender-Specific Strange Attractors Describe Human Brain Development during Childhood, Latency, Adolescence and Young Adulthood*

Harriet W. Hanlon[1,†] and John Dockery[2]
[1]Virginia Polytechnic and State University, Falls Church, Virginia, USA
[2]Fairfax County, Virginia, USA

Abstract

Time series of mean EEG coherence were used to track changes in synaptic potentials in a large sample of normal girls and boys, mapping the human cerebral neural networks emerging at 56 paired brain sites between birth and age 24 years. Development of neural networks proceeds in a sequence of synchronous and asynchronous growth periods suggesting that ontogenetic inputs establish the distinct stages of the life cycle. Networks have gender-specific signatures; each sex has local networks organized into complementary regional clusters. Accelerated regional networks emerge shortly after birth, while delayed networks emerge during the latency period. Accelerated networks have synchrony in growth and pruning in all local neural networks during childhood, asynchrony during latency and synchrony during adolescence. These gray matter expansions and contractions are for brain functions and skills primarily attributed to male hunters and female gatherers. Delayed regional networks have synchrony in local neural network growth and pruning during latency, asynchrony during childhood and adolescence and synchrony during young adulthood. Brain regions in these late

* This article was originally published in Chaos and Complexity Letters, volume 4 number 2 (2010).

† Corresponding Author's Email: hwhanlon@comcast.net.

In: Neuroscience and Technology Transform the Educational Ecosystem
Editors: Franco F. Orsucci and Nicoletta Sala
ISBN: 979-8-88697-157-6

developing networks sample the environment for a long period of time before plasticity is reduced. They are assumed to support more complex verbal and nonverbal reasoning tasks. Bifurcations or cusps ripple across all spatial gradients during latency marking the transfer of exuberant synchronized growth and pruning from the hunter/gatherer neural networks to the complex-reasoning neural networks. Each of the sexes' 56 neural networks has one or two discontinuities that can be cusp-fitted. The majority of networks align with only one regional cluster. Nonlinear analyses show that the sexes' neural networks develop as a sequence of low-dimensional strange attractors with age a surrogate for the underlying ontogenetic process. This study confirms that brain regions do not develop concurrently and that each sex has different critical periods for assimilating the culture in hunter/gatherer and complex-reasoning networks. The low fractal dimensions of the neural networks suggest genes rigidly program each stage of the life cycle for environmental input.

1. Introduction

Longitudinal and longisectional brain-mapping studies since 1999 add to existing evidence that the human cerebral cortex does not have concurrent development of neural networks from birth to late adolescence. Magnetic resonance image (MRI) studies by researchers at UCLA, McGill University and the National Institute of Mental Health (Thompson et al., 2000; Sowell et al., 1999; Giedd et al., 1999) show a gender-specific rosto-caudal wave of dramatic neural network growth and pruning in subjects aged 3 to 20 years. Previous cross-sectional MRI studies were not able to determine that (Giedd et al., 1999). The longitudinal MRI studies show this nonlinear emergence and provide definitive support for longisectional EEG coherence and phase studies that found neural networks emerge in cycles of growth and pruning that differ in the sexes and, within the sexes, differ in growth patterns across all spatial gradients. As with the MRI studies, these EEG patterns extend in time from birth to young adulthood (Thatcher, Walker and Giudice, 1987; Hudspeth and Pribram, 1990; Thatcher, 1992; Hanlon, Thatcher and Cline, 1999).

While understanding has been growing among neuroscientists for 20 years that synaptic and axonal connectivity are the instruments of computation, communication and connectivity among neural networks, only very recently have scientists shown how dramatically these neural connections change in both sexes over periods of time as short as one year (Thompson et al., 2000). Environmental and ontogenetic mechanisms responsible for the observed change in the numbers and/or strength of gray matter cortico-cortical connections include but may not be limited to the following: learning and culture; synaptogenesis; pruning of synaptic connections; axonal and dendritic sprouting; expansion of existing synaptic terminals; and changes in strength of neurotransmitter secretions during presynaptic and postsynaptic exchanges (Changeux, Heidmann and Patte, 1984; Kandel, 1985; Squire and Kandel, 1999).

While there is much behavioral, anatomical and physiological evidence that neural network functions change after late adolescence and throughout the life cycle (Blinkov and Glezer, 1968; Maccoby and Jacklin, 1974; Matsuura et al., 1985; Hudspeth and Pribram, 1990; Kimura, 1992; Hanlon, 1996), support for the observation that neural networks only gradually change or do not change at all after adolescence comes primarily from human and nonhuman primate postmortem counts of regional cortical synaptic density levels. Huttenlocher's human synaptic density studies (1999) found regional differences in synaptogenesis and in time envelopes needed for synaptic maturation and pruning to reach adult levels. Pruning synaptic density levels to the lower levels seen in adulthood varies by regions, with the visual cortex reaching adult levels by about age 10 years and the frontal cortex by late adolescence. While Huttenlocher's findings show support for the human brain not having concurrent development before adolescence, Goldman-Rakic, Bourgeois and Rakic (1997) found concurrent exuberant synaptogenesis in all brain regions of rhesus monkeys with density levels remaining high in all areas until puberty, after which all areas concurrently experienced attrition. With regard to synaptic maturation, neural network formation or hierarchical functional organization, Goldman-Rakic et al., suggested that the integrative nature of cortical neural networks requires that neural networks be distributed rather than hierarchical, that synaptogenesis be concurrent and that synaptic maturation and attrition be concurrent to insure retention of acquired experiences.

A flaw in extrapolating from post-mortem synaptic densities in rhesus monkeys and humans in early postnatal development to what is happening to synaptic networks in humans after adolescence is that postmortem counts cannot determine the cause of changes in synaptic potentials at connected brain sites. Potentials change when new synapses emerge, when existing synapses are eliminated or when secretions from neurotransmitters for existing connections increase or decrease. A neural network may reach a steady state in the number of connections and still be rewired; e.g., the neural network could shift support for specific connections by modifying the strength of neurotransmitters and supporting substructures or by emergence of new synapses as old ones are eliminated. Physiological measures are better suited than anatomical measures to elucidate dynamic changes throughout the life cycle.

Interest needs to shift to understanding the complex physiological processes involved in the dynamic reorganization of human cortical neural networks. The primary question will still be: do synaptic connections and supporting substructures mature until stability is reached in adolescence or do they change throughout the life cycle, with growth rate dependent on gender and life cycle stage. Stated another way: do gender-specific neural networks reach a steady state in early adolescence when cortico-cortical connections attrit to adult baseline levels or do gender-specific neural networks continue to rewire and reorganize even after adult baselines are reached. Specifically, do childhood, latency, adolescence, young adulthood, and later defined life stages represent different states of interconnectedness that emerge when ontogenetic inputs catalyze neural networks to accommodate experience-expected demands?

This study uses nonlinear analyses and cusp-fitting math models to confirm that all regions of the human brain do not develop concurrently and that each sex has a different ontogenetic timetable for emergence of their neural networks.

2. Method

The purpose of the present EEG study is to determine if postnatal development does proceed in distinct stages that are separated by discontinuities that can be cusp fitted. It brings nonlinear analysis methods to 56 time series of derived EEG coherence measures for girls and boys ranging in age from 2 months to 24 years to provide insights about cusp-like changes observed in sex development (Hanlon et al., 1999; Hanlon, 1996).

EEG coherence, a derived measure of wave synchrony of synaptic potentials at two spatially separated sites, is the measure of interest. Any coherence calculation involves converting EEGs from the time domain to the frequency domain. Coherence is a correlation measure in the frequency domain and is usually determined for the common frequency bands used by the human for internal brain communication; i.e., the alpha, beta, theta and delta bands. Coherence readings range from 0 to 1 and are usually reported as a percent. At least one minute of eyes-closed EEG is needed to precisely determine coherence at all paired neocortical sites in the brain (John, 1977); i.e., communication between and among brain sites is accurately determined with that amount of EEG assessment. A set of paired brain sites forms a local neural network; e.g., T3T5 is the local neural network of functional cortico-cortical connections between anterior temporal lobe site T3 and posterior temporal lobe site T5. A coherence reading of 0.35 for T3T5 means 35 percent of the synaptic potentials at the two sites are synchronized and in the same frequency band. A time series of coherence readings from a local network is constructed from EEG data collected over intervals of months and years. While a local neural network is a dynamic circuit, capable of some change throughout the life cycle, the circuit experiences its greatest amount of change during early postnatal development as it is established.

The initial gender EEG coherence study (Hanlon, 1994) found development in the 56 local neural networks proceeds in quasi-periodic cycles of growth and pruning with one or two cusp-like changes occurring in each network between birth and age 16 years. Each of the sexes' 56 neural networks included 64 time point samples, with median sample size of 16 for the 224 girls and 19 for the 284 boys. Each subject appeared in at most 4 consecutive time point samples of the oscillating development wave. The mean of the 56 female time series baselines was one percent lower than the male mean, with variance (peak-to-peak oscillations about the baseline) 88 percent greater. These differences support studies showing females have proportionately more gray matter and longer dendritic branches, while males have proportionately more white matter (Gur et al., 1995; Passe et al., 1997; Jacobs, Schall and Scheibel, 1993). The sexes' coherence time series correlated 0.190 in the left hemisphere and 0.130 in the right hemisphere, confirming very different postnatal patterns of coherence oscillations in the sexes' gray matter. Principal components analysis explained 94 percent of the variance in the 112 time series and, with no crossloading of neural networks, found nine clusters of similarly developing brain regions for each sex (called regional networks - see Figure 1). The sexes have complementary development of the regional neural networks established in childhood and latency. In childhood, girls favor functions linked with the left hemisphere and anterior frontal regions and boys favor functions linked with the right hemisphere and posterior occipital regions. In latency the sexes shift their focus, with girls now favoring functions linked with the right hemisphere and posterior occipital regions and boys favoring functions linked with the left hemisphere and anterior frontal regions. Both sexes develop the anterior right networks during latency. Another study (Hanlon, 1996) expanded the female 64 time point series by 12 time point samples and the male 64 time point series by 18 time point samples by adding EEG coherence data for 25 young adults between ages 17 and 24 years. This study confirmed that networks were still changing dramatically in the early twenties. For details on data collection, see Thatcher (1983; 1987); for details on gender differences, see Hanlon (1996; 1999).

For each of the sexes' 56 local neural networks, all of the following constructions or analyses were done:

- show a graph of the mean EEG coherence time series for the local network;
- determine the regional network cluster of local neural networks having similar development from birth to age 16- or 24-years;
- construct the strange attractor plots for the 16-year or 24-year time series and for the time periods (sub-stages) where the regional network showed synchrony;
- calculate the fractal dimensions for each of the time series used in strange attractor plots;
- determine the cusp fits for bifurcations in each local neural network's time series.

3. Results

All of the 112 time series were examined (56 for each sex) and all were found to have postnatal development that can be described by a strange attractor or sequence of strange attractors. Strange attractors are markers for systems where initial conditions are important for later functional outcomes and are typically of low correlation dimension and most often fractal. This section will examine in great detail 5 local neural networks for each sex. The networks selected are representative of brain development in both hemispheres and are useful for contrasting the sexes' developmental signatures. For each neural network, all or some of the following will be presented: the mean EEG coherence time series; the cluster of first derivative time series (regional neural network) with which the neural network has similar development from birth to age 16 or 24 years; the strange attractor plots for 16-year or 24-year time series and for at least one sub-stage of the time series; the fractal dimension for the 16- and 24-year time series; the fractal dimension for sub-stages representative of synchrony in the original time series; cusp fits for bifurcations in each time series; and cusp fits for sub-stages.

In the left hemisphere the neural networks examined include: T3T5, cortico-cortical integration of data from posterior and anterior temporal lobe sites T5 and T3, important for language production and concurrent discrimination; O1T3, cortico-cortical integration of visual inputs from occipital lobe site O1 at anterior temporal lobe site T3, important for functional tasks involving visual contrasts and graphic details; P3F7, cortico-cortical links between parietal site P3 and frontal lobe site F7, important for quick or suitable decision making. In the right hemisphere the neural networks examined include: T4T6, cortico-cortical links between posterior temporal site T6 and anterior temporal site T4, important for spatial navigation and recognition of nonverbal images and patterns; P4F8, cortico-cortical links between parietal site P4 and frontal lobe site F8, important for quick or suitable decision making. Sites were selected to represent clusters where one sex has earlier development than the other (females earlier in T3T5, males earlier in T4T6); where both sexes have early development (P3F7); where both sexes have late development (P4F8); and where the sexes have very different development trajectories as indicated by their regional networks and their strange attractors (O1T3).

4. Gender-Specific Regional Clusters of Neural Networks

Figure 1 shows head diagrams for the 9 clusters of regional neural networks for each sex, with each sex having brain regions with accelerated growth and other regions with delayed growth. Gould (1977; 1982) explains that accelerated growth or progenesis is needed for specie preservation and delayed growth or neoteny is needed for greater complexity. Clusters of EEG networks that show two periods of synchronized growth between birth and age 16 years have accelerated growth. The cognitive skills possible with accelerated neural networks have been classified by Kimura (1992) as the abilities needed by hunter/gatherers. Clusters that show only one period of synchronized growth between birth and age 16 years have delayed growth and support abilities needed for complex reasoning.

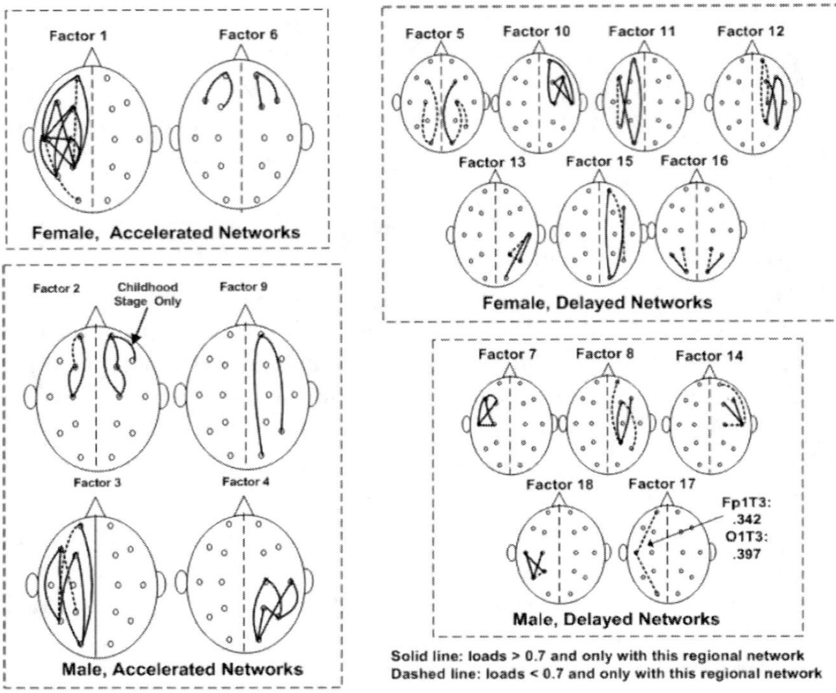

Figure 1. Gender-Specific Accelerated and Delayed Regional Networks.

Local neural networks in clustered regional networks concurrently experience one or two rapid changes in EEG coherence development by age 12 years, exhibited by phase-shifts in the coherence trajectories. Phase plots for each of the sexes' 56 neural networks can be classified as strange attractors as they do not converge to a point or limit cycle, but have definite structural properties (Ruelle, 1989). The easiest way to construct the strange attractor is with n-tuples of time delays of the original time series; alternate methods include n-tuples of the time series, its first derivative and succeeding derivatives (Ruelle, 1989). The majority of phase plots presented here are based on 3-tuple time delays with each attractor emerging as a compact set or sequence of compact sets in 3-space. A phase portrait type of phase plot is also presented for the sexes' T4T6 neural network because it better demonstrates visually the cusp being fitted. It consists of a 3-tuple with X equal to the raw data coherence time series, Y equal to its first derivative and Z equal to time in years. If the phase portrait is collapsed onto the XY plane its plot is almost congruent with the 2-tuple plot of time delays. All of the strange attractors for the sexes' 112 neural networks have low fractal dimensions, determined using software for analyzing chaotic data (Sprott and Rowlands, 1992). The software performs better with more points so interpolating two data points between each of the original data points expanded the time series with no effect on the growth and pruning peaks. The 64 time points were converted to 190 time points with the primary effect of smoothing the strange attractor.

5. Local Neural Networks from the Left Hemisphere

5.1. Local Neural Network T3T5

Figure 2 (female) and Figure 3 (male) show:

- T3T5 time series for mean EEG coherence;
- T3T5 strange attractors;
- Regional network containing first derivatives of T3T5 and local networks with similar development.

T3T5 is in an accelerated regional neural network for females (see Factor 1, Figure 1) and a delayed regional network for males (see Factor 18, Figure 1). The left temporal lobe is very important for concurrent discrimination and language processing. Females show one period of synchronized growth from birth to age 8 years and a second period of synchronized growth beginning at age 13 years; males show only one period of synchronized growth beginning around age 7 years and ending around age 11. Phase shifts or bifurcations are present in both sexes' mean EEG coherence development. Table 1 lists the correlation or fractal dimensions for the T3T5 time series and for sub-stages when the neural network experienced robust growth. A sub-stage was defined as the set of time points from the onset of synchronized growth within the associated regional neural network to the onset of asynchrony. The embedding dimension is a 5- or 10-dimensional sphere that contains the 3-dimensional strange attractor. In most neural networks, the fractal dimensions for each attractor had minimal positive slopes with embedding dimensions between 2 and 10.

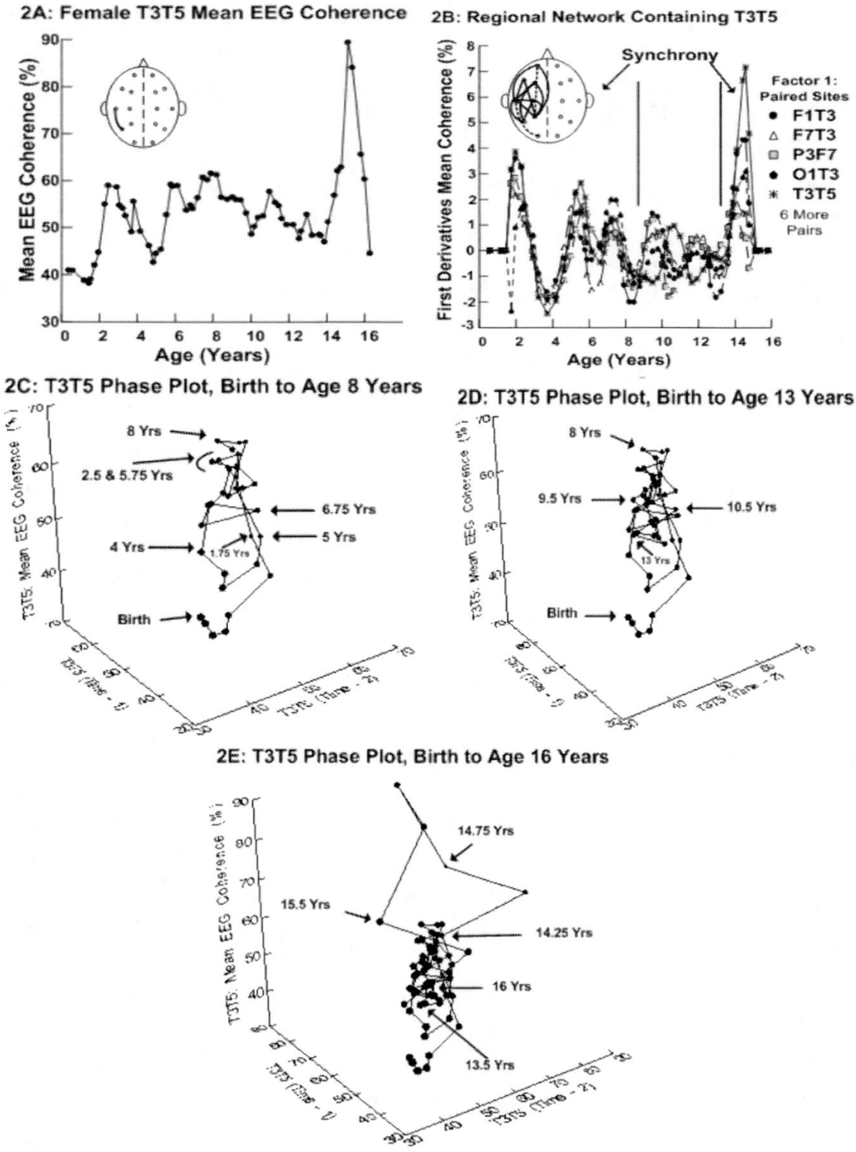

Figure 2. Female Local Network T3T5 (2A), Regional Network Containing T3T5 (2B) and Phase Plots for T3T5 Strange Attractor (2C, 2D and 2E).

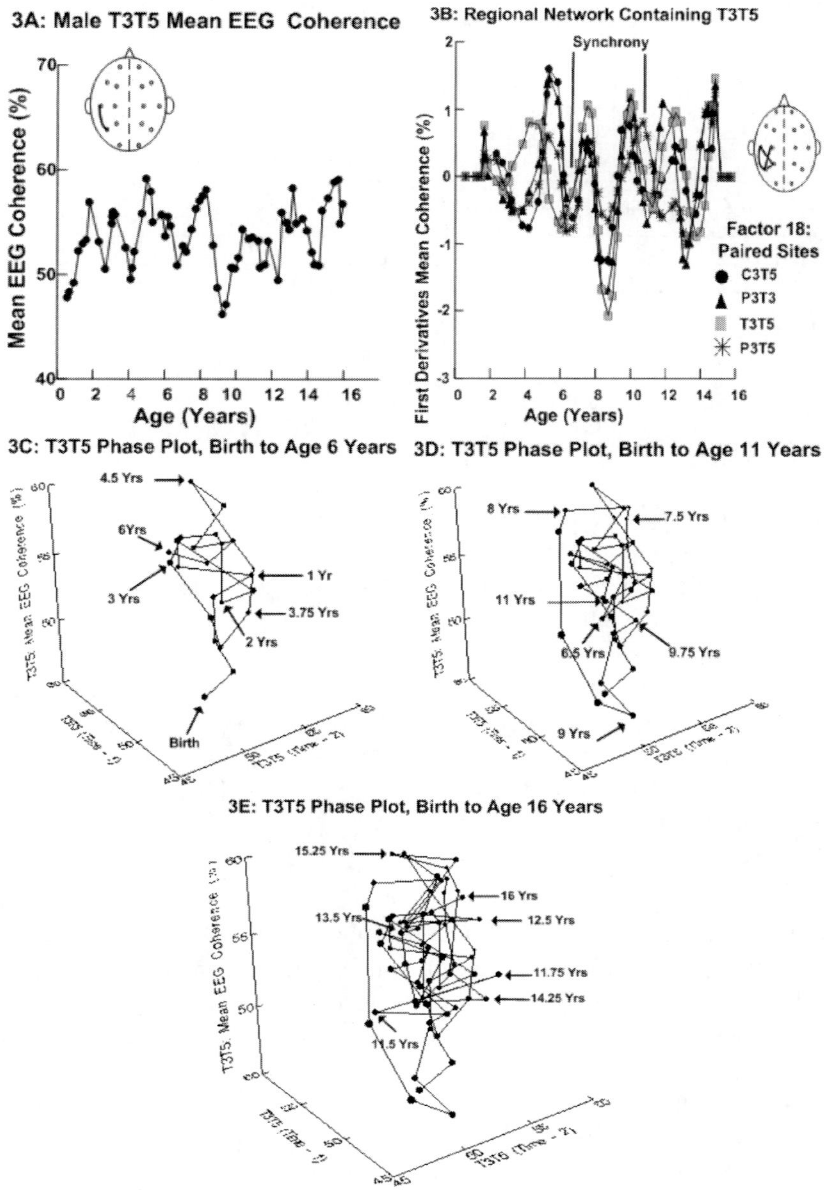

Figure 3. Male Local Network T3T5 (3A), Regional Network Containing T3T5 (3B) and Phase Plots for T3T5 Strange Attractor (3C, 3D and 3E).

Table 1. Female and male T3T5 fractal dimensions

T3T5 Mean EEG Coherence Time Series	Female: fractal dimension		Male: fractal dimension	
	Embedding Dimension: 5	Embedding Dimension: 10	Embedding Dimension: 5	Embedding Dimension: 10
Birth to Age 16 Yr	2.482	3.635	2.848	4.721
Birth to Age 8 Yr	2.016	2.331	-----	------
Age 7 to 11 Yr	------	------	2.301	2.500
Age 13 to 16 Yr	1.156	1.373	------	------

5.2. Local Neural Network O1T3

Figure 4 (female) and Figure 5 (male) show:

- O1T3 time series for mean EEG coherence;
- O1T3 strange attractors;
- Regional network containing first derivatives of O1T3 and local networks with similar development.

O1T3 is in an accelerated regional network for females (see Factor 1, Figure 1) and a delayed regional network for males (see Factor 17, Figure 1). The time series were extended to age 24 years for both sexes to compare attractors and determine if a second cusp could be captured in the late developing male neural network. O1T3 represents the visual pathway for orthographic details like letters and numbers. While female O1T3 has low loading on Factor 1 (see Figure 1), it loads on no other regional neural network. It experiences two periods of robust growth by age 16 years with significant pruning during the asynchronous period from age 8 to 12 years. Male O1T3 loads very weakly with Fp1T3 on Factor 17 (see Figure 1), with synchronized growth only from age 13 to 16 years. Since all neural networks in both sexes have synchronized growth throughout the brain around age 16 years, it appears that the male's O1T3 neural network has unique development. Prior to age 9 years it primarily experiences a steady decline in coherence, indicating the number or strength of cortico-cortical connections is decreasing. The phase plots show male development from birth to age 16 years as a sequence of two strange attractors, with the first established from birth to age 9 years and the second between 9 and 14 years. At age 15 years the data shift back to the initial attractor.

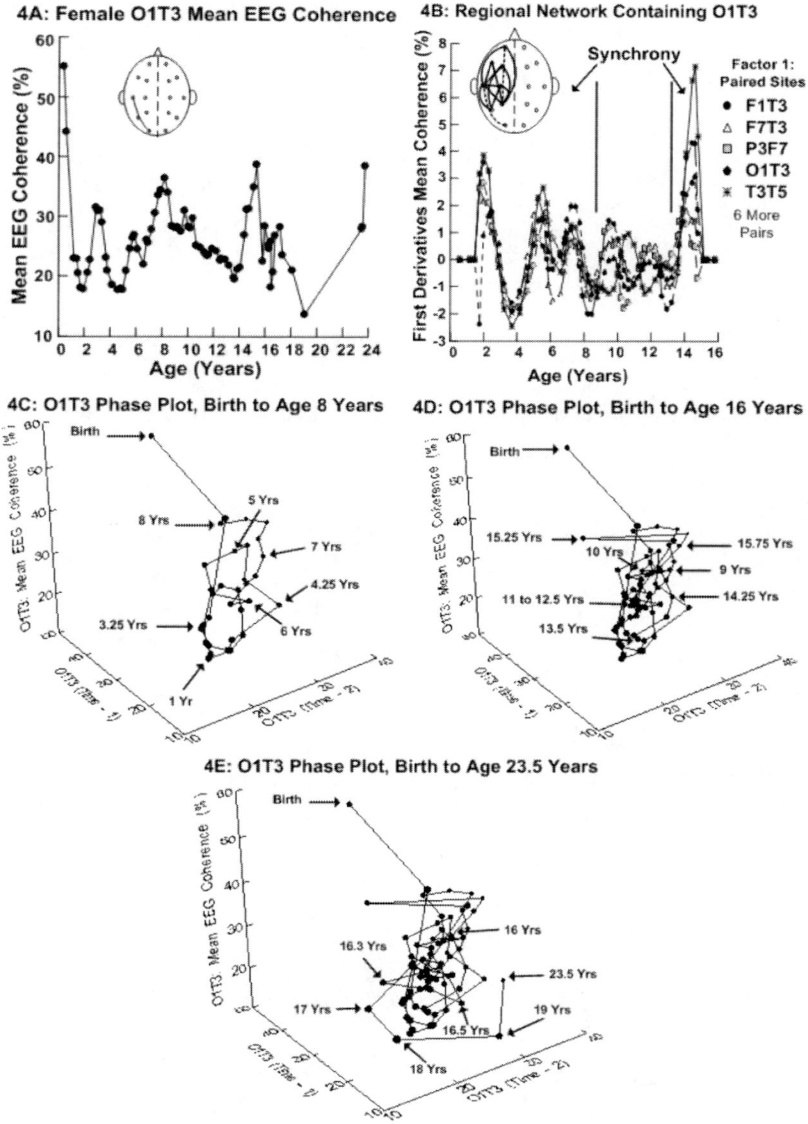

Figure 4. Female Local Network O1T3 (4A), Regional Network Containing O1T3 (4B) and Phase Plots for O1T3 Strange Attractor (4C, 4D and 4E).

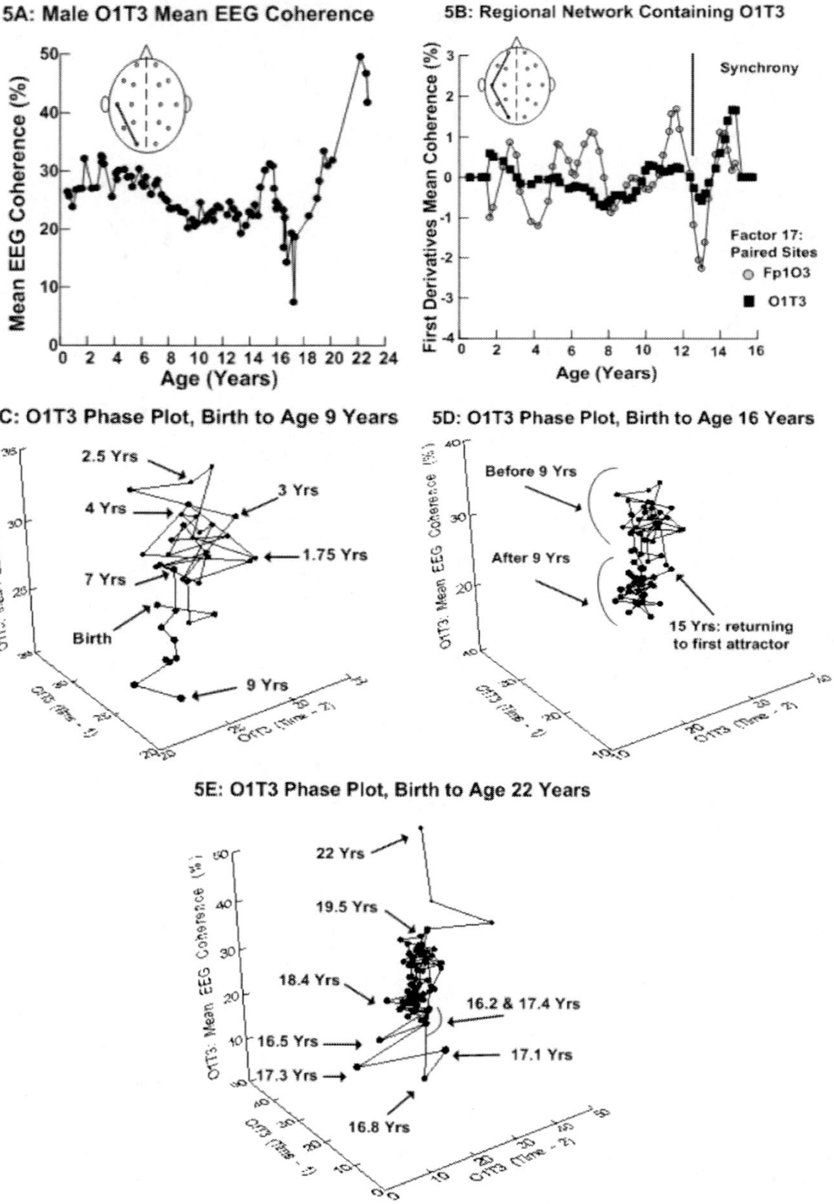

Figure 5. Male Local Network O1T3 (5A), Regional Network Containing O1T3 (5B) and Phase Plots for O1T3 Strange Attractor (5C, 5D and 5E).

Table 2. Female and male O1T3 fractal dimensions

O1T3 Mean EEG Coherence Time Series	Female: fractal dimension		Male: fractal dimension	
	Embedding Dimension: 5	Embedding Dimension: 10	Embedding Dimension: 5	Embedding Dimension: 10
Birth to Age 24 Yr	2.288	2.816	2.720	4.013
Birth to Age 8 Yr	1.314	1.668	------	------
Age 9 to 16 Yr	------	------	3.209	3.797
Age 13 to 16 Yr	2.204	1.436	------	------

Table 2 lists the fractal dimensions for O1T3 from birth to age 24 years and for sub-stages when the neural network experiences robust growth.

5.3. Local Neural Network P3F7

Figure 6 (female) and Figure 7 (male) show:

- P3F7 time series for mean EEG.coherence;
- P3F7 strange attractors;
- Regional network containing first derivatives of P3F7 and local networks with similar development.

P3F7 is in an accelerated regional network for females (see Factor 1, Figure 1) and an accelerated regional neural network for males (see Factor 3, Figure 1). This neural network involves transfer of perceptual information to the orbital frontal lobes. In both sexes it clusters on the factor that explains the most variance in development of left hemisphere neural networks in early postnatal development. Female P3F7 clusters with language processing and concurrent discrimination networks; male P3F7 clusters with visual tracking and targeting networks. Each of these neural networks participates in two periods of robust growth by age 16 years. For both sexes, the phase plot for the strange attractor has two basins of attraction. Table 3 lists the fractal dimensions for P3F7 from birth to age 16 years and for sub-stages when the neural network experiences robust growth.

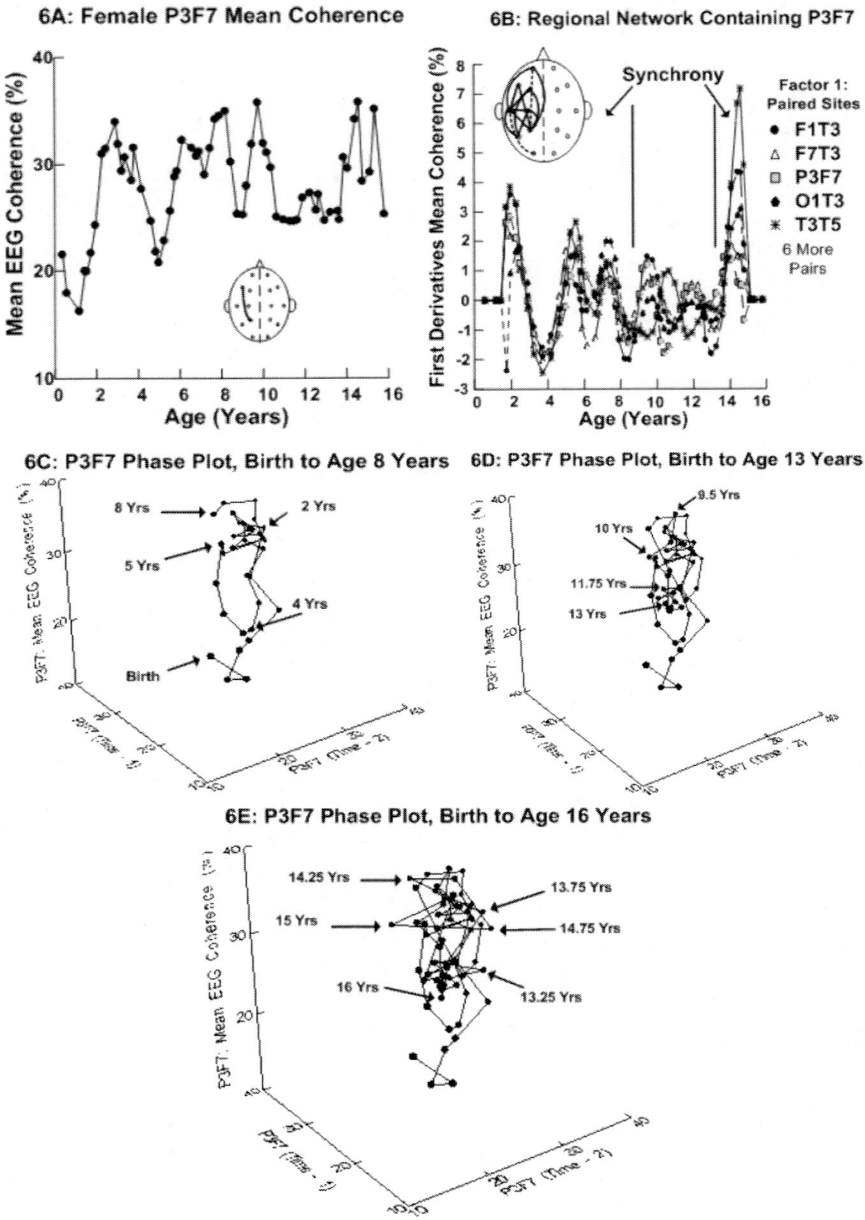

Figure 6. Female Local Network P3F7 (6A), Regional Network Containing P3F7 (6B) and Phase Plots for P3F7 Strange Attractor (6C, 6D and 6E).

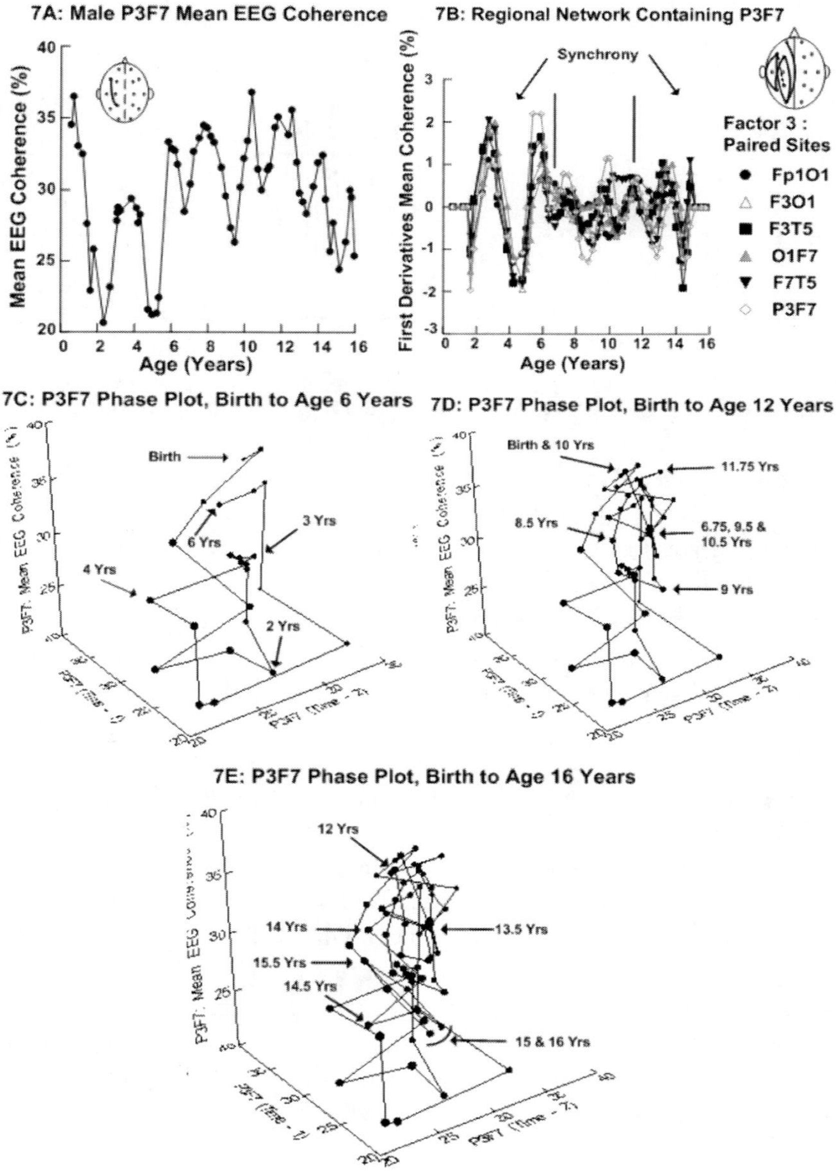

Figure 7. Male Local Network P3F7 (7A), Regional Network Containing P3F7 (7B) and Phase Plots for P3F7 Strange Attractor (7C, 7D and 7E).

Table 3. Female and male P3F7 fractal dimensions

P3F7 Mean EEG Coherence Time Series	Female: fractal dimension		Male: fractal dimension	
	Embedding Dimension: 5	Embedding Dimension: 10	Embedding Dimension: 5	Embedding Dimension: 10
Birth to Age 16 Yr	2.500	3.699	2.502	3.015
Birth to Age 8 Yr	2.784	2.744	------	------
Birth to Age 6 Yr	------	------	1.392	1.235
Age 13 to 16 Yr	1.298	2.130	------	------
Age 11 to 16 Yr	------	------	1.879	1.960

6. Local Neural Networks from the Right Hemisphere

6.1. Local Neural Network T4T6

Figure 8 (female) and Figure 9 (male) show:

- T4T6 time series for mean EEG coherence;
- T4T6 strange attractors;
- Regional network containing first derivatives of T4T6 and local networks with similar development.

Figure 10 (both sexes) shows phase portraits that better illustrate the cusps in the sexes' T4T6 time series. Its 3-tuples consist of age, mean EEG coherence reading and first derivative of mean EEG coherence reading.

T4T6 is in a delayed regional neural network for females (see Factor 13, figure 1) and an accelerated regional neural network for males (see Factor 4, figure 1). The time series were extended to age 24 years for both sexes to compare attractors and determine if a second cusp could be captured in the late developing female neural network. The right temporal lobe is very important for concurrent discrimination of touch with vision and for integration of spatial information needed for navigation. Males show one period of synchronized growth from birth to age 6 years and a second period of synchronized growth beginning at age 11 years; females show only one short period of synchronized growth beginning around age 8 years and continuing until age 12 years. Phase shifts or bifurcations are present in both sexes' mean EEG coherence development. Table 4 lists correlation or fractal dimensions for the T4T6 time series and for sub-stages when the neural network experiences robust growth.

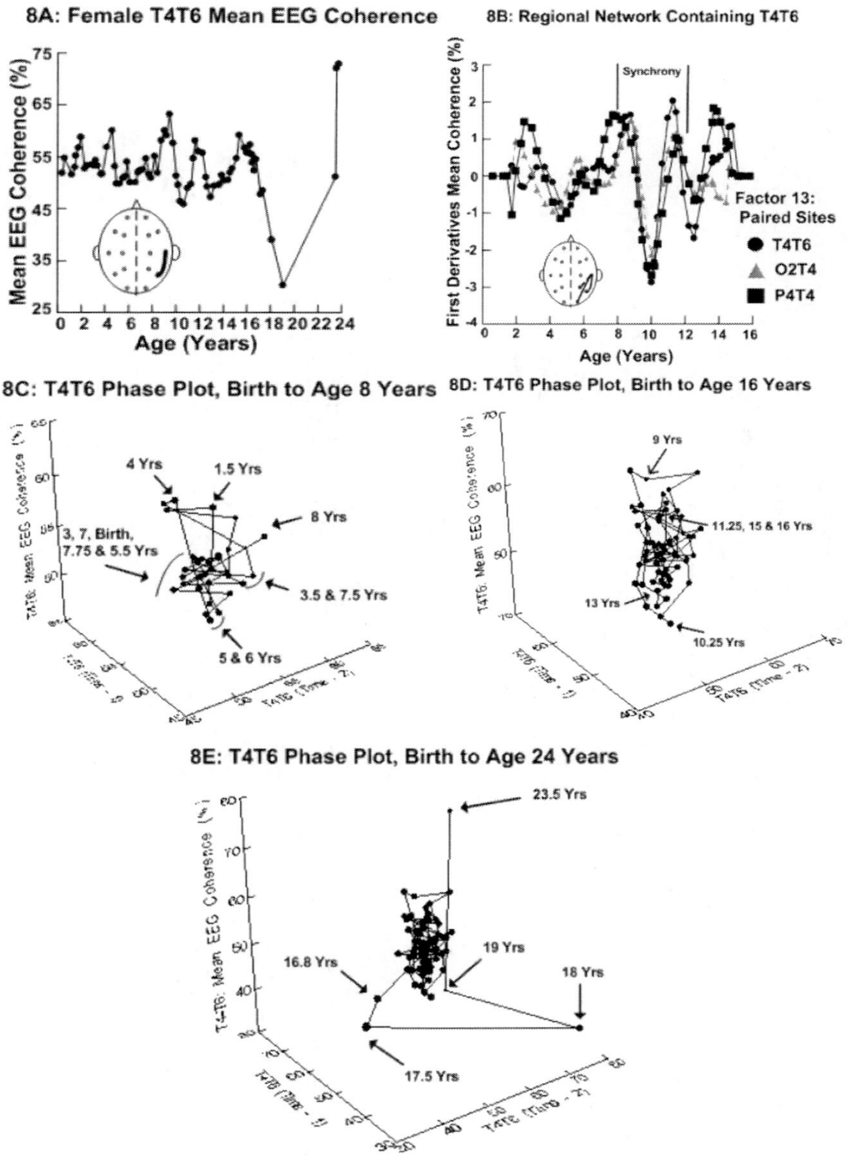

Figure 8. Female Local Network T4T6 (8A), Regional Network Containing T4T6 (8B) and Phase Plots for T4T6 Strange Attractor (8C, 8D and 8E).

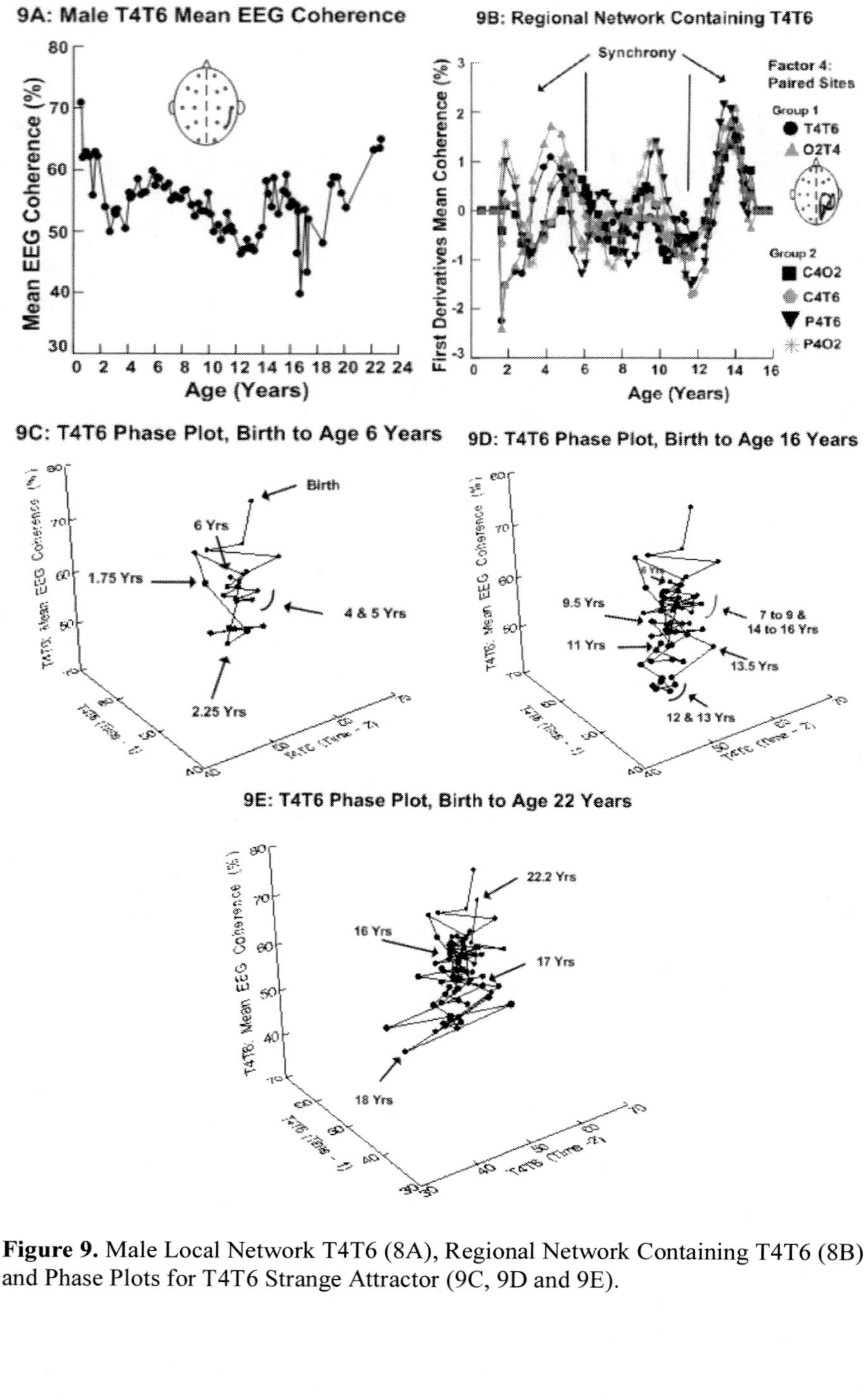

Figure 9. Male Local Network T4T6 (8A), Regional Network Containing T4T6 (8B) and Phase Plots for T4T6 Strange Attractor (9C, 9D and 9E).

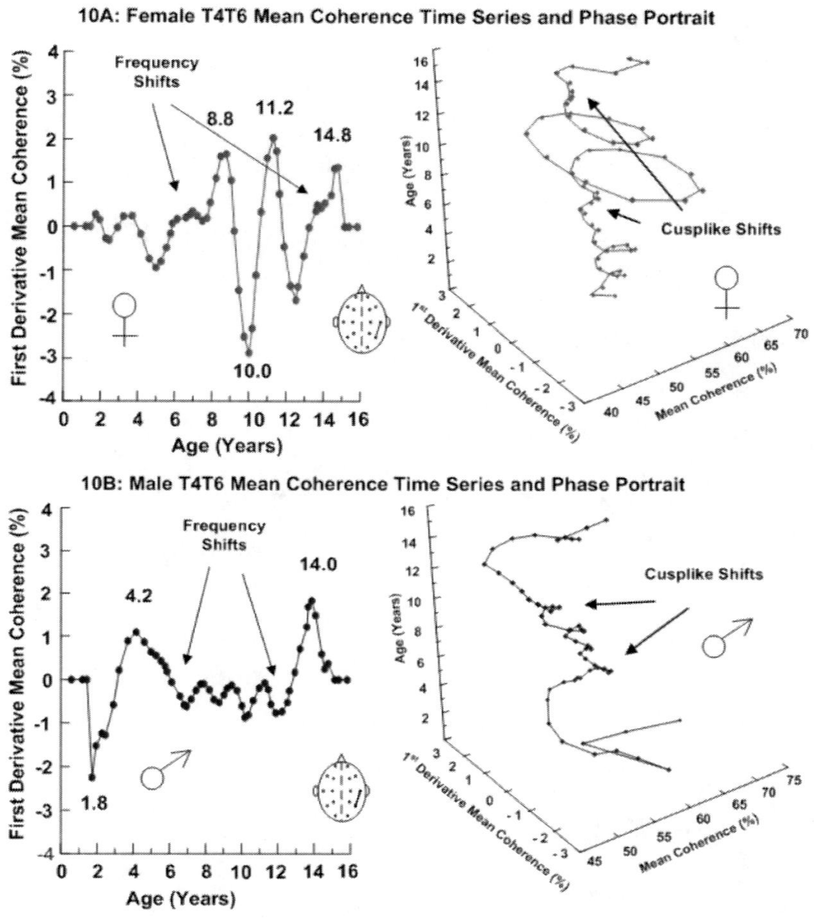

Figure 10. Female (10A) and male (10B) Local Network T4T6 First Derivate Mean Coherence Time Series and 3-Dimenstional Phase Portrait (modified, Hanlon: 1996).

Table 4. Female and male T4T6 fractal dimensions

T4T6 Mean EEG Coherence Time Series	Female: fractal dimension		Male: fractal dimension	
	Embedding Dimension: 5	Embedding Dimension: 10	Embedding Dimension: 5	Embedding Dimension: 10
Birth to Age 24 Yr	2.745	3.440	2.645	3.959
Birth to Age 6 Yr	------	------	1.723	2.653
Age 8 to 12 Yr	2.002	2.081	------	-----
Age 11 to 16 Yr	------	------	2.317	2.521

6.2. Local Neural Network P4F8

Figure 11 (female) and Figure 12 (male) show:

- P4F8 time series for mean EEG.coherence;
- P4F8 strange attractors;
- Regional network containing first derivative of P4F8 and local networks with similar development.

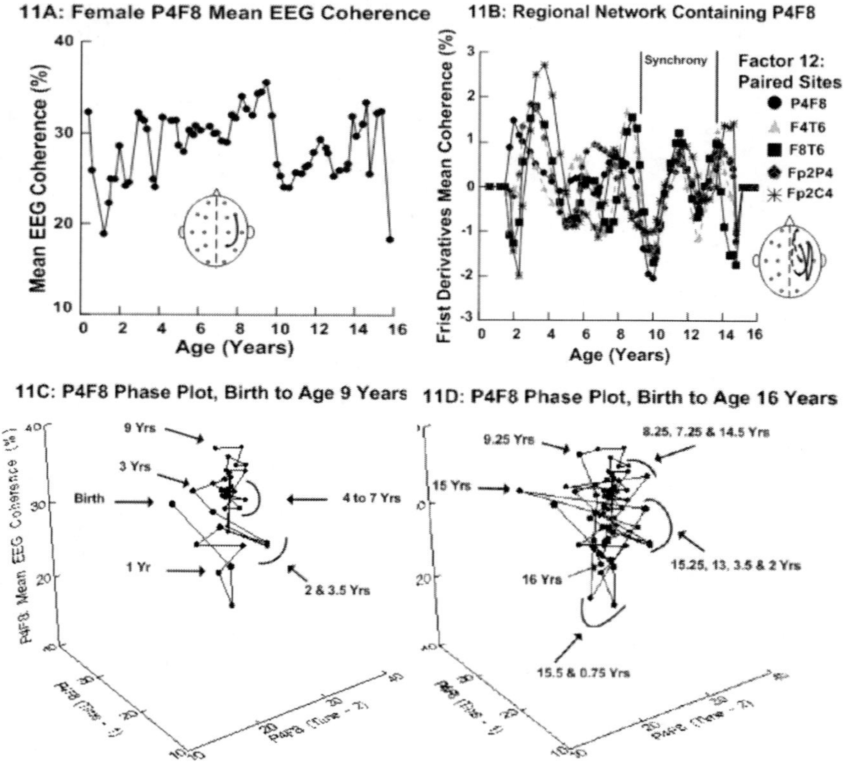

Figure 11. Female Local Network P4F8 (11A), Regional Network Containing P4F8 (11B) and Phase Plots for P4F8 Strange Attractor (11C and 11D).

P4F8 is in a delayed regional neural network for females (see Factor 12, Figure 1) and a delayed regional neural network for males (see Factor 8, Figure 1). In both sexes P4F8 has robust growth during the asynchronous period from birth to age 9 years, with the axis about which the growth and pruning cycles oscillate showing a steep increase across the period. The phase shift at age 9 years (see Figures 11A and 12A) includes a dramatic drop in these baselines. Table 5 lists correlation or fractal dimensions for the P4F8 time series and for sub-stages when the neural network experiences robust growth.

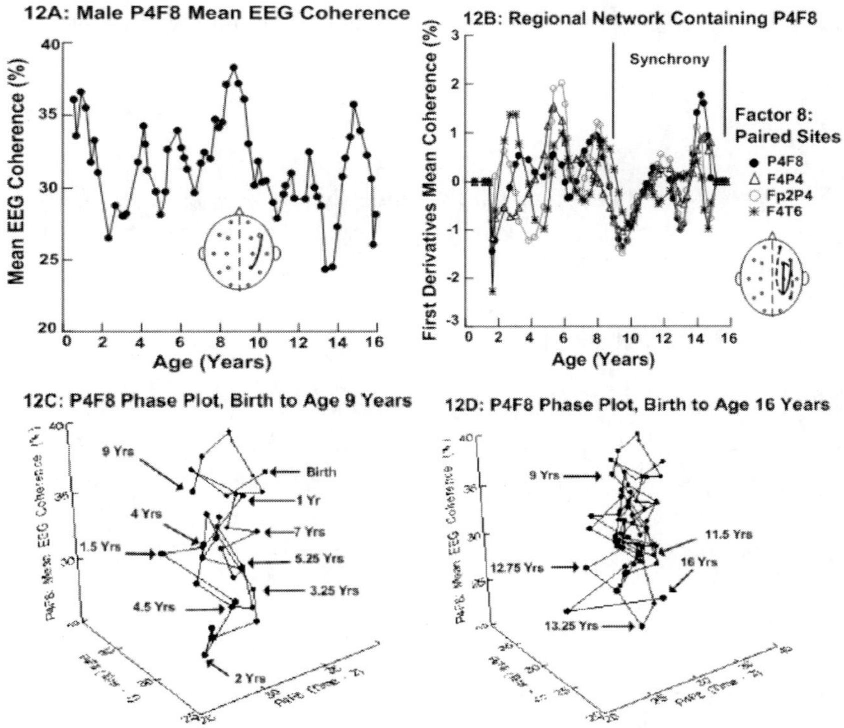

Figure 12. Male Local Network P4F8 (12A), Regional Network Containing P4F8 (12B) and Phase Plots for P4F8 Strange Attractor (12C and 12D).

Table 5. Female and male P4F8 fractal dimensions

P4F8 Mean EEG Coherence Time Series	Female: fractal dimension		Male: fractal dimension	
	Embedding Dimension: 5	Embedding Dimension: 10	Embedding Dimension: 5	Embedding Dimension: 10
Birth to Age 16 Yr	2.290	2.895	2.678	4.249
Age 9 to 16 Yr	1.483	1.753	2.548	3.079

7. Fitting the Neural Network Data to a Cusp Manifold

Visual inspection of the sexes' T4T6 neural network data in Figure 10 phase portraits reveals dramatic cusps. In order to test for the existence of a cusp, a fitting program written by Loren Cobb [1983; 2006] was employed. Cobb's program attempts to fit available data to the following hypothesis:

$$0 = \alpha + \beta z - \delta z^3 \tag{1}$$

where $z = (y - \gamma)$. If we designate the independent or control variables as x_j $(j = 1,v)$, and cite y as the dependent or behavior variable, then the conditional density of y given $x_1,\ldots, x_v$ is

$$f(y|x) = \exp[\, \Psi + \alpha z + \beta z^2/2 - \delta z^4/4 \,] \tag{2}$$

with

ψ = constant with respect to y, and
$\alpha = a_0 + a_1{*}x_1 + \ldots + a_v{*}x_v,$
$\beta = b_0 + b_1{*}x_1 + \ldots + b_v{*}x_v,$
$\gamma = c_0 + c_1{*}x_1 + \ldots + c_v{*}x_v$.

Fits for each sex's 56 neural networks were possible only with age as the dependent variable y and $v = 1$ with x_1 being the coherence time series data from various paired sites in the brain (local neural network). The Cobb program uses a maximum likelihood function to generate all coefficients for equations (1) and (2). Not all of the neural networks examined yielded a fit for the 64 time points from birth to age 16 years although a fit was always possible if the data were divided into two increments of birth to age 8 (or 9) years and age 8 (or 9) to 16 years. Fits with 76 or 82 time points were less frequent suggesting the existence of more than one cusp in the passage between birth and age 20+ years. Some experimentation, not reported here, was also done with age as the control variable and the coherence time series and its derivative as the dependent variables.

Three conditions were necessary and sufficient to confirm that human brain development for a specific neural network followed a cusp catastrophe model (Cobb, 2006).

- First, the null hypothesis that the coherence data satisfies a linear model has to be rejected; i.e., the coefficients generated for equation (1) could not yield a response surface Y that is flat; this would occur if δ was not statistically different from 0.
- Second, the coefficients α, β and δ have to be statistically different from 0 and δ has to be positive; i.e., the coefficients generated for equation (1) yield a response surface Y that contains a smooth pleat called the bifurcation zone (see Figure 13A which depicts a general cusp manifold). Figure 13B shows that the system modeled may be in one of two stable states. However, if the system falls from one state to another, say from the upper sheet at point 2 through the cusp to the lower sheet at point 3, there is no immediate return path. A capsizing ship is a good example of this kind of catastrophe event. Up to a certain point small corrections serve to keep the boat upright. Beyond that point major effort is required. In Figure 13B, traveling from the upper sheet to the lower sheet through point 1 avoids the bifurcation zone and indicates that the system can best be described by the linear model.

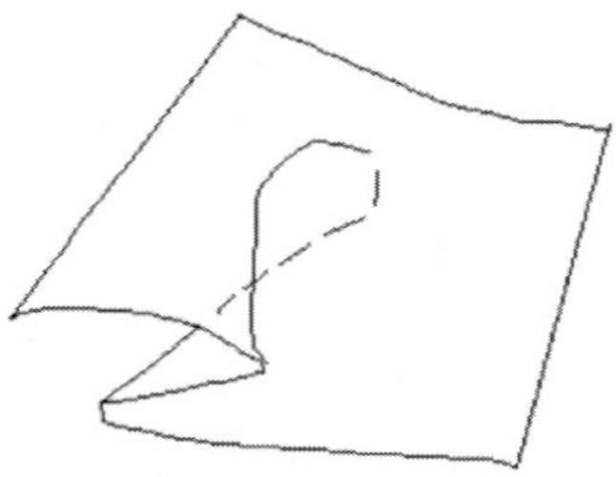

Figure 13A. Generalized cusp manifold.

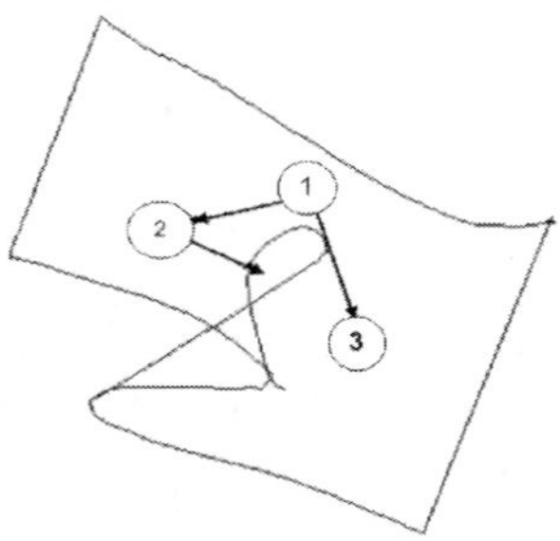

Figure 13B. Two possible paths on the manifold from point 1 to point 3.

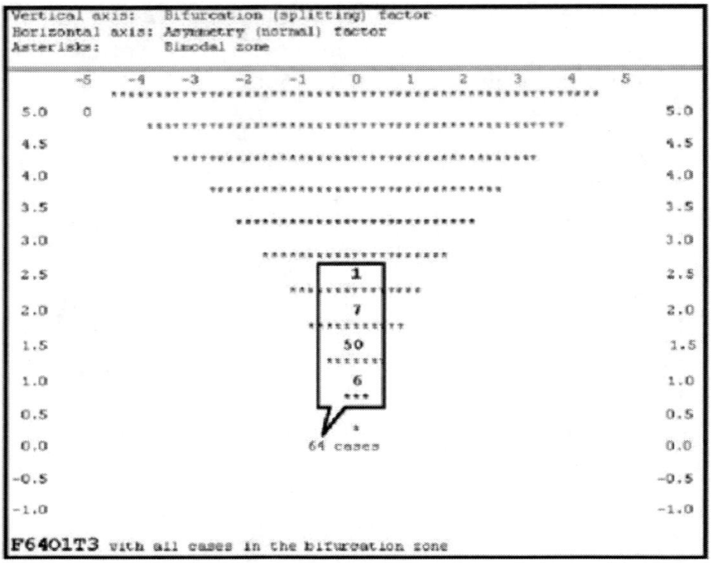

A. Top down view of cusp for female O1T3 (64 time points; numerals indicate no. of cases occurring at the specified location).

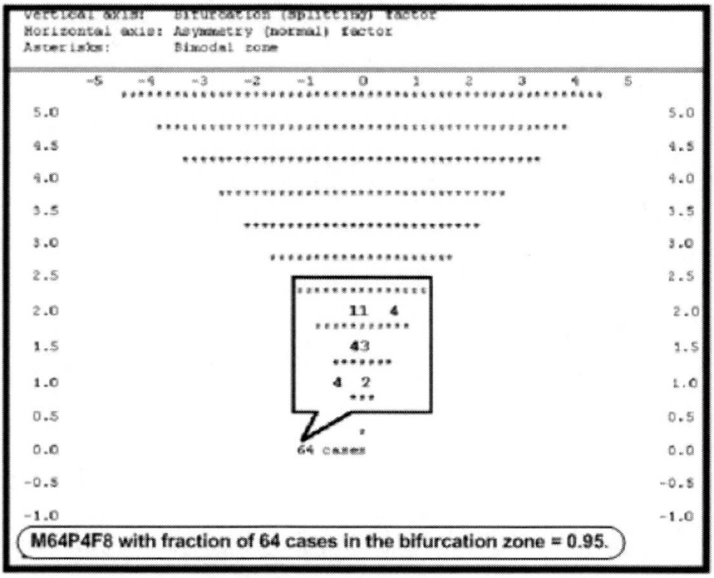

B. Top down view of cusp for male P4F8 (64 time points; numerals indicate no. of cases occurring at specified location).

Figure 14. Examples of time points tightly clustered on bifurcation axis.

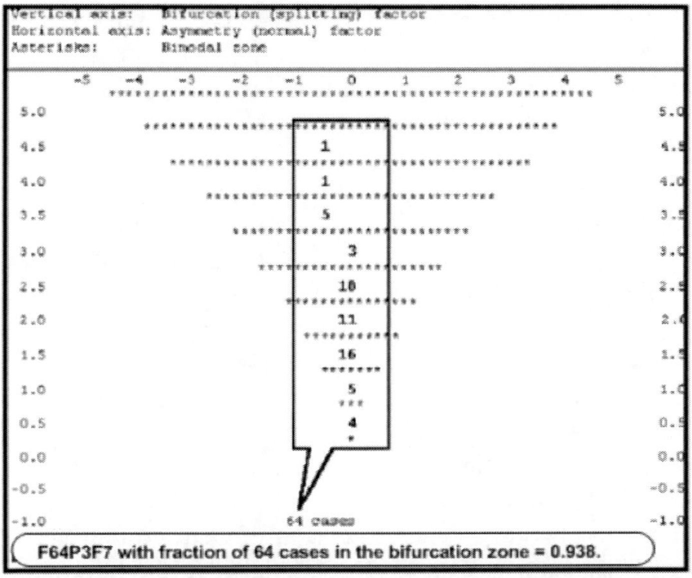

A. Top down view of cusp for female P3F7 (64 time point; numerals indicate no. of cases at specified location).

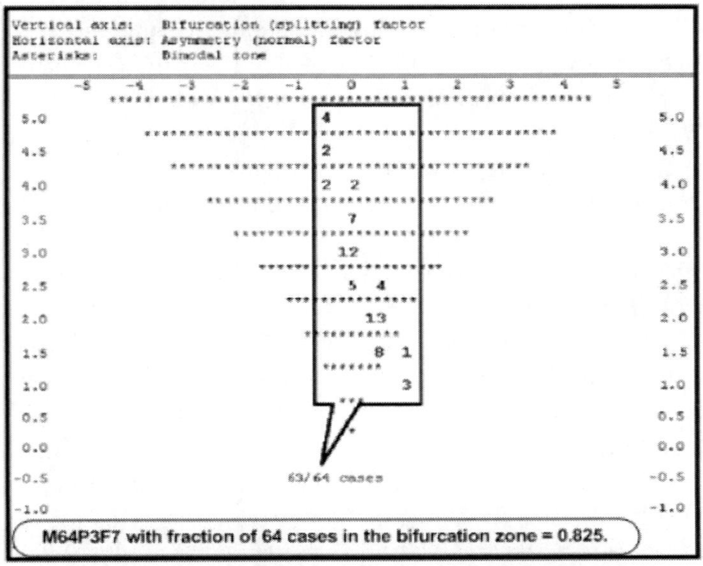

B. Top down view of cusp for male P3F7 (64 time point; numerals indicate no. of cases at specified location).

Figure 15. Examples of time points with great dispersion on bifurication axis.

- Third, at least 10 percent of the data for the control variable must be trapped in the pleated area of the cusp (the bifurcation zone). Figures 14 and 15 show female and male local neural networks with more than 87 percent of the coherence data in the bifurcation zone.

As data passes through the bifurcation zone, it is positioned in the bimodal zone on three axes. The two in the plane are based on the control variables, with asymmetry on the horizontal axis and bifurcation on the vertical axis; the axis perpendicular to the plane is the behavior variable. Figures 14 and 15 show a top down view of cusp manifolds with the bimodal region indicated by asterisks. The numbers embedded in the bimodal region show the number of data entries at that location irrespective of their location along the behavior axis. Some fits, as in Figure 14A (female O1T3) and 14B (male P4F8), were concentrated in a small cluster. Others, as in Figure 15A (female P3F7) and 15B (male P3F7), were strung out along the bifurcation axis. The program prints out the location of all entries in terms of their location as a function of asymmetry, bifurcation and a triplet. The latter is the node-antinode-node combination resulting from the three roots of cubic equation (1).

One could interpret cusp fits for female and male neural network P3F7 (Figure 15) as showing transitions that are patiently ongoing in time in the neural network. The points are distributed along the bifurcation axis to values of +5 while in Figures 14A and 14B (female O1T3 and male P4F8) they all lie within values of +2 units. In the former, it suggests that some brain regions linger in one stage as long as possible even as they are beckoned to move onto the next stage; in the latter, it suggests that other brain regions move quickly from one stage to the next.

In virtually all the fits to the neural network cusps, the delay convention was the fit of choice. This indicates that data transitions from one sheet of the manifold to the other only after all support for the initial site disappears. In contrast the Maxwell cusp convention describes a system where passage from one sheet of the manifold to the other is done as quickly as possible. For most of the neural networks the δ coefficient for the cubic term of equation (1) being fitted to the Maxwell model was negative, indicating no support in the coherence data for this fit. While the R^2 for the coefficients for equation (1) linear fits were low, the Maxwell fit was often lower or nonexistent. Table 6 lists the results of the fitting program for the sexes' 5 neural networks, with sub-stages considered for some networks. All cusp fits in the table were determined using the delay convention model. The following equation shows the fit in z for female network O1T3:

$$0 = (-0.004 - 0.09x_1) + (1.514 + 0.245x_1)z - 1.415z^3,$$

where $z = (y - 0.005 + 0.044x_1)$.

Table 6. Cusp program fits for male and female brain development

Time Series: Birth to Age 16 Years								
Local Neural Networks	Male				Female			
	Time Points	Linear R2	Cusp R2	Fit	Time Points	Linear R2	Cusp R2	Fit
O1T3	64	--	--	N	64	0.001	0.714	Y
T3T5	64	0.044	0.885	Y	64	0.191	0.813	Y
T4T6	64	--	--	N	64	0.004	0.647	Y
P4F8	64	0.047	0.700	Y	64	0.000	0.768	Y
P3F7	64	0.022	0.605	Y	64	0.055	0.745	Y
T4T6 Cusp Fits for Shorter Periods								
Birth- 9yrs	35	0.146	0.709	Y	34	0.029	0.714	Y
14-22yrs	26	0.202	0.766	Y	26	-	-	N
9yrs-24yrs	47	-	-	N	34	-	-	N
O1T3 Cusp Fits for Shorter Periods								
Birth - 9yrs	35	0.131	0.882	Y	34	-	-	N
4-14.5yrs	26	0.202	0.733	Y	43	0.000	0.700	Y
9yrs- 24y/rs	47	0.318*	0.695	Y	30**	0.003	0.582	Y

* 0.462 (Maxwell) – one of the few cases where the Maxwell fit was better than the linear fit.
**To 16 years.

Conclusion

With reference to the information from the analysis of the attractors and their dimensions, a complex process is underway. The strange attractor plots demonstrate that in female accelerated neural networks P3F7, O1T3 and T3T5 restrictions on structure are established by the end of childhood. For example, female P3F7 establishes its outer boundary by age 7 years with two sub-attractor regions contained within, with each enhanced and revisited often between age 7 and 16 years. Similarly, the plots for the male accelerated neural networks P3F7 and T4T6 show outer boundaries established by the end of childhood; e.g., male T4T6 establishes its outer boundary by age 6 years with one sub-attractor region established by age 2 years and the other by age 4. Late developing female neural networks T4T6 and P4F8 and male neural networks T3T5 and P4F8 take to the end of the latency period to establish the outer boundary and seem to contain only one very diffuse attractor basin. Male neural network O1T3 spends from birth to age 8 years in one attractor basin, from age 9 to14 years in a second attractor basin, and from age 15 to 24 years expanding the outer boundaries of the two basins. Since this neural network establishes two distinct basins by age 16 years, it may be misclassified as a delayed network. This development will be of particular interest for the subset of boys who are classified as "probable dyslexic" but show improvement on tests for visual details and begin reading after age 9 years (Rumsey, 1998). Males may use the first basin more for functions related to visual contrasts and the second for visual details such as color and letters.

The fractal dimensions are low for all the neural networks, but lower in number and closer to zero slope when a subset of the time series is taken that represents a period in which the neural network has synchronized growth with its regional network. Selecting this subset of time points is equivalent to taking the points from the most concentrated portions of the attractor basin. When periods of asynchronized growth with the regional network are examined the fractal dimension for the asychronized portion of the neural network's development is higher than for the synchronized period, but lower than the dimension for the entire 16- or 24-year periods. Selecting this subset of time points is equivalent to taking the time points that are either in transit between basins or expanding the structural limits of the strange attractor's boundary. These differences suggest that ontogenetic inputs are stronger in initiating synchronization than asynchronization.

In the epoch of childhood individual neural networks vary in the structural limitations placed on their cycles of growth, assimilation, and pruning. In the latency period when neural networks in the delayed regional networks get the ontogenetic green light to establish their functions, the hunter/gatherer dominated net must at once cooperate in assimilating the higher reasoning neural networks but not at the expense of existing distributed functions that were costly to construct and are most likely still useful. With each succeeding period of growth and pruning, it is usually the case that more than one focus occurs for the attractor. These are age related. One basin appears before others, but the original is usually revisited from time to time. What can be expected in the cusp fits? If age is accepted as a surrogate for some physical process which is a *f(t)*, then the development seems clearly to be separated into epochs of synchronized growth followed by periods of adjustment to the new structure. The cusps should mark establishment of the new structure as a new attractor basin, whether within the original boundary or in a new expanded boundary. Hence, neural networks in accelerated networks should demonstrate periods in which at least two cusps could be fitted, while neural networks in delayed networks should demonstrate a period in which at least one cusp could be fitted. Table 6 indicates some success in doing this. At least one cusp was determined for all female neural networks between birth and age 16 years and for male neural networks T3T5, P4F8 and P3F7. Where fits could not be obtained for the 16-year time period for male O1T3 and T4T6, the longer data set for the 24-year time period was examined and split into three time domains. The results are sensitive to the choice of interval but suggest that both neural networks have two cusps. This agrees with the strange attractor plots and with the regional neural network plots. The longer time series were also examined for the same sites for the females. Two cusps were determined for O1T3 and one for T4T6, which also agrees with strange attractor plots and regional neural network plots.

It should also be noted that the fitting program treats but one of ten possible catastrophe surfaces. These are mostly the time dependent cusps. In some of these the lip of the cusp moves in time even though the process does not move along a trajectory. It is as if the environment has shifted making the old location disappear. Manifolds of higher dimension than the cusp exist. For example the butterfly has four control variables. In one of its 3-dimensional projections it looks like the cusp with an intermediate sheet. This would be the case for multiple cusp transitions and would be true for brain development only if an intermediary growth state eventually disappeared. While the evidence is limited, the strange attractor pattern of often revisiting earlier basins would seem to eliminate this occurrence. The revisiting also may insure that acquired experiences are retained and refreshed. There remains the identification of the bifurcation axis and the asymmetry axis with physical processes such as ontogenetic or environmental inputs.

The stages of childhood, latency, adolescence and young adulthood represent sequential states of development in the distributed neural networks of the human brain. The stages can be described by the sequence of synchronous/asynchronous development in mean EEG coherence time series of the regional neural networks. The stages are separated by discontinuities that can be cusp fitted. Distinct brain regions can be described by strange attractor patterns that differ in the sexes and in both change across time. The sexes favor early development of neural networks that support specie preservation, later development of neural networks for higher-level thinking. At each of these stages, the sexes favor robust development of complementary brain regions. Ontogenetic input can be observed in the strange attractor plots and in the low dimensional correlations of the compact sets, suggesting that initial conditions are determined for each stage by the DNA and that rewiring of cortico-cortical connections occurs throughout the observed period from birth to age 25. Strange attractor patterns that emerge in the early twenties do not suggest that the dynamic process is about to end.

References

Blinkov, S. M. & Glezer, I. I. (1968). *The human brain in figures and tables*. Plenum Press: New York.

Changeux, J-P., Heidmann, T. & Patte, P. (1984). Learning by selection. In P. Marler & H. S. Terrance (Eds.) *The biology of learning.* New York: Springer- Verlag.

Cobb, L., (1983). *A Pascal computer program to fit a cusp hypothesis using a maximum likelihood method.* Department of Biometry, Medical University of South Carolina, Charleston, S.C.

Cobb, L. (2006). Website: www.aetheling.com. *Aetheling Consultants.* Carbondale, Colorado 81623.

Goldman-Rakic, P. S., Bourgeois, J. P. & Rakic, P. (1997). Synaptic Substrate of Cognitive Development. In, N. Krasnegor, G. Lyon & P. S. Goldman-Rakic (Eds.) *Development of the prefrontal cortex.* Baltimore, MD: Paul H. Brookes.

Gur, Ruben C., Lyn Harper Mozley, P. David Mozley, Susan M. Resnick, Joel S. Karp, Abass Alavi, Steven E. Arnold, and Raquel E. Gur. (1995). Sex differences in regional cerebral glucose metabolism during a resting state. *Science.* 267, 528-531.

Giedd, Jay N., Jonathan Blumenthal, Neal O. Jeffries, F. X. Castellanos, Hong Liu, Alex Zijdenbos, Tomáš Paus, Alan C. Evans, and Judith L. Rapoport. (1999). Brain development during childhood and adolescence: a longitudinal MRI study. *Nature Neuroscience.* 2 (10), 861-863.

Gould, S. J. (1977). *Ontogeny and phylogeny*. Cambridge, MA: Harvard University Press.

Gould, S. J. (1982). Change in developmental timing as a mechanism of macroevolution, in *Evolution and development.* J. T. Bonner (Ed.)

Hanlon, H. W. (1994). *Differences in female and male development of the human cerebral cortex from birth to age 16*, U.M.I. Dissertation Information Service. #9507750.

Hanlon, H. W. (1996). Topographically different regional networks impose structural limitations on both sexes in early postnatal development. In K. Pribram & W. King (Eds), *Learning as self-organization.* (pp. 311-376). Mahwah, NJ: Erlbaum.

Hanlon, H. W., Thatcher, R. W. and Cline, M. J. (1999). Gender differences in the development of EEG coherence in normal children. *Developmental Neuropsychology.* 16 (3), 479-506.

Hudspeth, W. J. & Pribram, K. H. (1990). Stages of brain and cognitive maturation. *Journal of Educational Psychology.* 82 (4), 881-884.

Huttenlocher, P. R. (1999). Dendritic and synaptic development in human cerebral cortex: time course and critical periods. *Developmental Neuropsychology*. 16 (3), 347-349.

Jacobs, B., Schall, M. & Scheibel, A. B. (1993). A quantitative dendritic analysis of Wernicke's area in humans -- II. gender, hemispheric and environmental factors. *Journal of Comparative Neurology*. 327, 97-111.

Kandel, E. R. (1985). Synapse formation, trophic interactions between neurons, and the development of behavior. In E. R. Kandel & J. H. Schwartz (Eds.), *Principles of neural science*. New York: Elsevier Science Publishers.

Kimura, D. (1992). Sex differences in the brain. *Scientific American*. (September), 119-125.

Maccoby, E. E. & Jacklin, C. N. (1974). *The psychology of sex differences*. Stanford, CA: Stanford University Press.

Matsuura, M. et al. (1985). Age development and sex differences of various EEG elements in healthy children and adults -- quantification by a computerized wave form recognition method. *Electroencephalography and Clinical Neurophysiology*. 60, 394-406.

Passe, T. J., Rajagopalan, P., Tupler, L.A., Macfall, J. R. & Krishnan, D. R. R. (1997). Age and sex effects on brain morphology. *Progress in Neuro-Psychopharmacology and Biological Psychiatry*. 21, 1231-1237

Ruelle, D. (1989). *Chaotic evolution and strange attractors*. Cambridge University Press.

Rumsey, J. *Presentation on learning disability profiles in boys*. Krasnow Institute. George Mason University, Spring, 1998.

Sowell, E., Thompson, P. M., Holmes, C. J., Jernigan, T. L. & Toga A. W. (1999). In vivo evidence for post-adolescent brain maturation in frontal and striatal regions. *Nature Neuroscience*. 2 (10), 859-861.

Sprott, J. C. & Rowlands, G. (1992). *Chaos Data Analyzer*, Physics Academic Software. North Carolina State University, Raleigh, NC.

Squire, L. R. & Kandel, E. R. (1999). Memory from mind to molecules. *Scientific American Library*. New York: W H Freeman. .

Thatcher, R. W. (1983). Hemispheric EEG asymmetries related to cognitive functioning in children. In E. Perecman (Ed), *Cognitive Processing in the Right Hemisphere*. New York: Academic Press.

Thatcher, R. W., Walker, R. A. & Giudice, S. (1987). Human cerebral hemispheres develop at different rates and ages. *Science*. 236, 1110-1114.

Thatcher, R. W. (1992). Cyclic cortical reorganization during early childhood. *Brain and Cognition*. 20, 24-50.

Thompson, P. M., Giedd, J. N., Woods, R. P., MacDonald, D., Evans, A. C. & Toga, A. W. (2000). Growth patterns in the developing brain detected by using continuum mechanical tensor maps, *Nature*. 404, 190-193.

Section 2. Technology

Chapter 9

Extended Reality in Education

Nicoletta Sala*
Institute for Complexity Studies, Italy
Institute for Scientific and Interdisciplinary Studies (ISSI), Switzerland
Institute for Arithmetic Physics (IRFIA), Switzerland

Abstract

The transfer of knowledge is an important feature in the educational environments and in the learning. It represents one base for our society. In the era of digital devices, there are many opportunities to enable better learning with technology. In particular, extended reality (XR) is a term that includes virtual reality (VR), augmented reality (AR), mixed reality (MR), and their derived virtual learning environments (VLE) seem to be the natural next step for the evolution of education. This work describes how XR can transform the way in which educational contents are delivered in these first decades of 21st century.

Keywords: augmented reality, education, cross reality, extended reality, mixed reality, virtual learning environment, virtual reality

1.Introduction

About two centuries ago, the Swiss pedagogue Johann Heinrich Pestalozzi (1746-1827) observed that students learn best through physical activity and if they use their senses (Pestalozzi, 1803).

---

* Corresponding Author's Email: nicolettasala@alice.it.

In: Neuroscience and Technology Transform the Educational Ecosystem
Editors: Franco F. Orsucci and Nicoletta Sala
ISBN: 979-8-88697-157-6

More recently, the educational environments find in the new technologies and in the new media of communication the ways to improve the learning paths. For example, virtual reality (VR), Augmented reality (AR), and mixed reality (MR) can stimulate the senses of the students. In particular, involving them in learning activities with a high degree of participation, where the students play active roles. These technologies can also help to create virtual learning environments which help to improve the learning.

We can refer to VR, AR and MR introducing the term: extended reality (XR, or abbreviated as ER) also known as cross reality. Medium.com (2018) gives to XR the following definition: "It refers to all real-and-virtual combined environments and human-machine interactions generated by computer technology and wearables."

This work describes the use of XR in the school where the integration can be possible between the old traditional didactic methods with the modern methods, based on multimedia technologies, and new learning environments. The work is organized as follows. First paragraph introduces virtual reality, its short history and applications in educational fields.

The same organization for the second and the third paragraph where augmented reality and mixed reality are described. Future trends of extended reality are in the fourth paragraph. Last paragraph is dedicated to the conclusions.

2. Virtual Reality

Virtual reality (VR) is a technology which involves information technology, computer graphics and electronics, and it gives its users the illusion of being immersed in a computer-generated virtual world with the ability to interact with it using special devices (Sala, 2021). The first use of the term "virtual reality" was in the title of a paper written in 1987 by Yaakov Garb. For this author, VR is the capability to represent the world with visual symbols (Garb, 1987).

Two years later, American computer scientist Jaron Lanier used the term virtual reality to specify the world of computer technology (Heilbrun and Stacks, 1989, p. 108). In this interview, Lanier defines the VR as "a world without limitation, a world as unlimited as dreams. It's also a world that's shared" (Heilbrun and Stacks, 1989, p. 109).

More recently, the Encyclopædia Britannica (2021) describes VR referring "the use of computer modeling and simulation that enables a person to interact with an artificial three-dimensional (3-D) visual or other sensory environment" (Lowood, 2021).

Table 1. The three primary requirements of VR

Immersion	Interaction	Visual realism
Immersion refers to a realistic feeling that allows users to have exposure to a virtual world. There are three categories of immersion: tactical, strategic, and narrative.	Interaction is a kind of action that occurs as two or more objects have an effect upon one another. It is the natural interaction between the users and the virtual scenes.	Visual realism provides an accurate representation of the virtual world using computer graphics tools and virtual scenarios.

Table 2. Virtual reality classification (Riva, 2006)

Type	Features
Desktop VR	It is a solution for virtual reality low cost, which uses a computer monitor as a display to provide graphical interface for users. The interaction with the virtual world is not high, and it can be made via mouse or joystick, and it does not require any expensive hardware or software, and it is also relatively easy to develop.
Fully Immersive VR	This is the name given to a virtual environment in which the user has the illusion to be fully immersed within it. This illusion is created using immersive output devices (for example, stereoscopic goggles) and a system of tracking to have the correct correspondence between user's movements and the feedback in the virtual environment.
CAVE (Cave Automatic Virtual Environment)	It is a room where its walls are typically made up of projection screens, where a world generated by computer is projected on the walls. Its name is also a reference to the allegory of the Cave in Plato's *Republic* in which a philosopher contemplates perception, reality, and illusion. This solution is particularly suggested for collective VR experience because different people can share the same experiences at the same time.
Telepresence	This term is used to describe a set of technologies, such video, audio, and other interactive elements, that permit the users to feel or appear as if they are present in a location in which they are physically not located. Users can influence and operate in a world that is real but in a different location. This technology is used as a collaborative tool. Telepresence and videoconferencing are different. Telepresence offers face-to-face interactions between the people in the meeting through the transmission of life-size, high-definition images and audio.
Augmented Reality (AR)	It is a direct or indirect view of a real-world environment which elements are augmented (or supplemented) by computer-generated sensory input such as graphics, sound, and video. For example, the user's view of the world is enriched by virtual objects, usually to provide information about the real environment. Augmentation is in real-time. Typical hardware components for augmented reality are: processor, input devices, display, sensors, and smartphone.

The three primary requirements of a VR system were defined by Rosenblum & Cross (1997). They are: immersion, interaction, and visual realism. The next Table 1 resumes these features.

Riva (2006) classifies virtual reality in five categories (desktop VR, fully immersive VR, CAVE, telepresence, augmented reality). Table 2 resumes this classification and its features.

VR can be also classified according to its methods of display. In detail:

- immersive VR which involves a high degree of interactivity and high cost of peripheral devices, for example the head mounted displays (an example in Figure 1a); and

- non-immersive VR is often called desktop VR and it is in the form of a windows into a virtual world displayed on a computer's monitor (an example in Figure 1b).

The participation, the sense of reality, and the degree of involvement in the virtual worlds created by virtual reality technologies are possible with the use of different devices. In particular, input devices, output devices, graphic rendering and database construction for virtual objects. In the details:

- The input devices which report, in real time, the position and the movements of the users in the virtual worlds. Input devices can include trackers, keyboards, mouse (2D or 3D), and gloves.
- The output devices (visual, aural, and haptic) give the users the illusion to be immersed in the virtual environments.
- The graphic rendering system generates the virtual scenarios and the virtual environments; and
- The database construction and virtual object modelling software realize virtual scenarios and detailed and realistic models of the virtual world. In particular, the software handles the geometry, texture, intelligent behavior, and physical modelling of any object included in the virtual world.

Figure 2 shows an example of VR I/O devices: virtual reality headset and wired gloves; Figure 3 resumes the components of VR systems (Whyte, 2002).

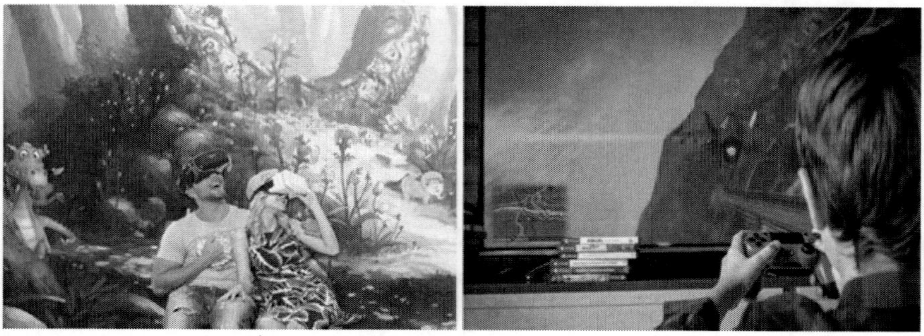

a) b)

Figure 1. Immersive VR a). Non immersive VR b).

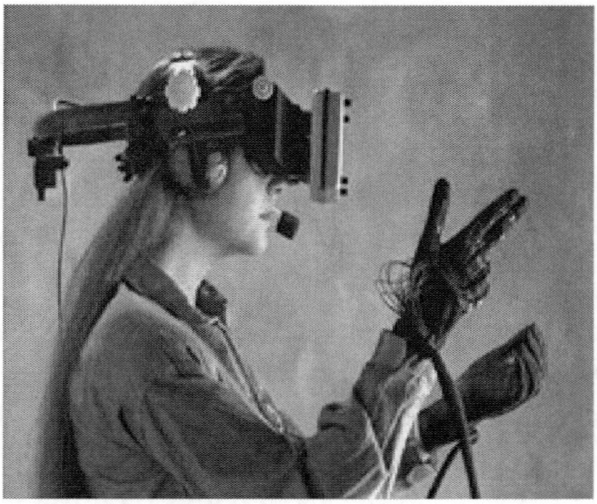

Figure 2. Virtual reality devices: a woman wearing a head-mounted display incorporating Pop Optics goggles developed by NASA's Ames Research Center, and wired gloves. The goggles are now displayed in the Dulles Annex of the National Air and Space Museum of the Smithsonian Institution.

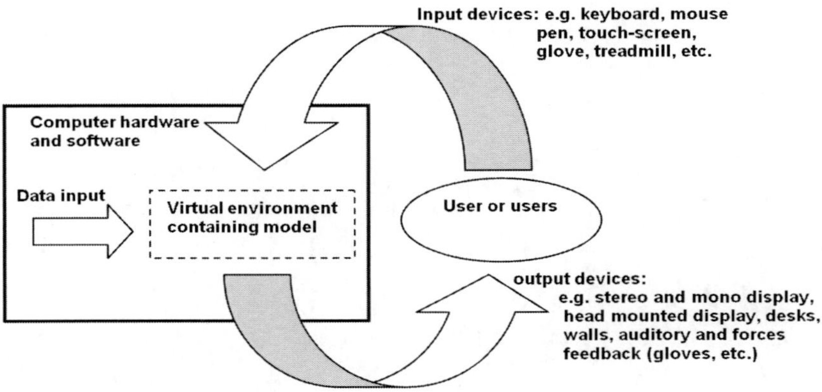

Figure 3. The components of a VR systems.

Educational theory and cognitive science support the exploration of VR as an educational tool. Many researchers believe that VR technology offers strong benefits that can support education, for example to facilitate constructivist activities (Winn, 1993).

Using constructivist theory, Byrne (1996) created a virtual chemistry world to encourage students to learn by exploring and interacting with the information. Instead of sitting in a classroom and passively viewing images of atomic orbitals in a traditional lesson, students can place electrons into an atom and see the atomic orbital appear as the electron buzzes. In this constructivist approach, the immersive virtual world was created by high school students involved in the project. Thus, the role of the students was active in their learning process. Byrne affirmed that the results of her study have not shown VR to be superior to other methods of instruction; but interactivity, an important VR's feature, could be relevant for the learning (Byrne, 1996). This case study emphasized that VR does not furnish only passive interactions, but its reconstruction of reality is a model where users can act and interact. Users behave as in real world. This important feature overcomes the inherent limitations of perception, which should be applicable only to objects physically perceptible.

The realism in virtual worlds is another important feature because helps the sense of immersion of the users.

In 2002, Sala et al. described the connections between VR, fractal geometry, and computer graphics to realize a set of virtual worlds, where the students also generated buildings, trees, mountains, lakes, and special effects using fractal algorithms (Sala et al., 2002). Figure 4 shows an example of fractal trees generated by Lindenmayer systems (L-systems). This set of fractals can be used to create digital sceneries in computer graphics environments (Sala, 2008).

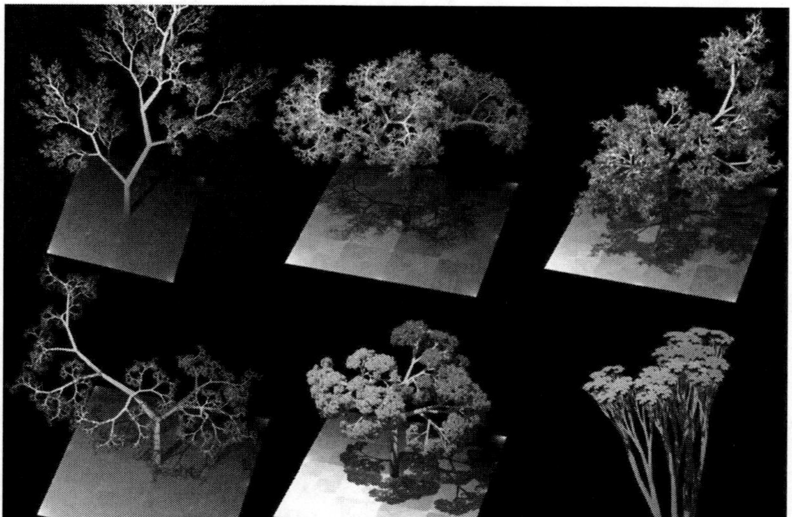

Figure 4. Fractal trees created with L-systems which can used in virtual environment.

In 2005, Sala and Sala analyzed the contribution of multimedia technologies and VR in university courses of mathematics and information technology to a faculty of architecture in Switzerland. In this educational project, the term "virtual reality" has been used to cover both immersive and non-immersive VR. The technology was used first to help architecture students to visualize in 3D, since this is arguably the most difficult part of understanding architecture. The undergraduate students used the VR technologies in different ways, for example as media to create virtual towns and virtual worlds also in the world wide web (Sala & Sala, 2005). For example,

- to observe, to create, and to manipulate the geodesic domes,
- to create virtual objects and virtual polyhedra using VRML (Virtual Reality Modeling Language),
- to observe and to interact the molecules of carbon (C60 and C70) from the different points of view,
- to study and to observe the symmetry present in the crystals, and
- to create virtual mountains, virtual trees and virtual buildings using fractal algorithms.

In this study, the students' roles were active because they designed virtual territories and virtual scenarios using computer graphics tools and fractal algorithms, in agreement to the results of other researches (Guérin et al., 2002; Sala, 2009; 2016).

Over the years, the evolution of technology helped to lower the cost of VR interfaces. In this way, it was easier to integrate VR into educational processes. For example, recent studies introduce complex medical database visualization, 3D visualization of anatomy for medical education, telepresence surgery, VR surgical simulators, rehabilitation, and virtual prototyping of surgical equipment and operating rooms (Ghezzi & Corleta, 2016, Latifi & Latifi, 2018, Bhattarai et al., 2019, Shakya et al., 2019, Jin et al., 2021, Xia & Lu, 2021).

Other important application field is in the Computer Numerical Control (CNC). In this educational environment VR helps to teach to the students how to set-up, maintain, operate and dismantle machining tools that are controlled by computers, before entering a real laboratory equipped with real machine tools, for example, lathes and milling machines (Tsai, Kao, & Lee, 2012).

Other application is to use VR in a Mini CNC machine assembly simulator (Malik & Hady, 2021).

These approaches allow to the students to use real machine tools safely, after training with virtual reality environment.

During these decades, VR technology has applications across many academic disciplines and has the potential to contribute to student centered, experiential learning opportunities (Hurrell & Baker, 2021).

3. Augmented Reality

Augmented reality is a direct or indirect view of a real-world environment whose elements are augmented (or supplemented) by computer-generated sensory input such as graphics, sound, and video. For example, the user's view of the world is supplemented with virtual objects, usually to provide information about the real environment. Augmentation is in real-time (Sala, 2021).

Encyclopedia Britannica defines augmented reality as "a process of combining or 'augmenting' video or photographic displays by overlaying the images with useful computer-generated data." (Hosch, 2021).

In this way, the environment is "augmented" by more information.

The term "augmented reality" was coined in 1990 by Thomas Caudell and David Mizell referring on a technology to support an industrial process at Boeing, in particular to describe how the head-mounted displays that electricians used when assembling complicated wiring harnesses worked. (Höllerer & Feiner, 2004).

AR is a direct or indirect view of a real-world environment with elements augmented by computer-generated sensory input such as graphics, sound, and video. For example, the user's view of the world is enriched by virtual objects. An example of AR is shown in Figure 5.

Among the peculiar characteristics of AR we can indicate the possibility of interaction with virtual objects and the versatility of its use in relation to the objectives to be achieved (communication, education, marketing).

To realize an environment based on AR are necessary: Hardware components for AR. They include: a processor, a display, sensors, and input devices.

Augmented Reality technology is not a new technology. It has been used in fields such as: medicine, military, robotic, manufacturing, engineering design, consumer design, psychological treatments, etc.

One of the first use of AR in education was in the last year of the 20th century.

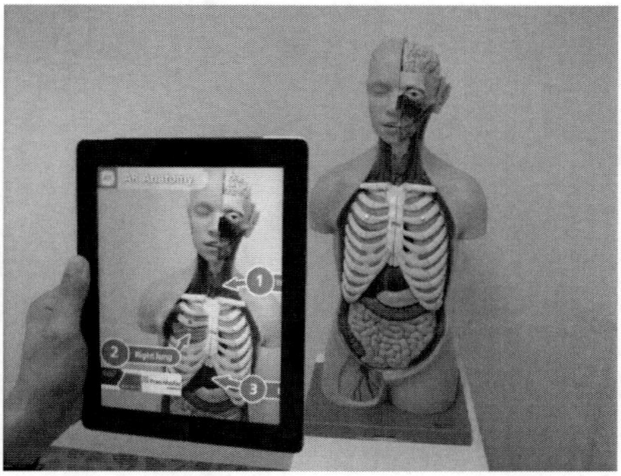

Figure 5. An example of augmented reality.

In 1996, Schmalsteig et al. presented the StudierStube project, an example of collaborative learning with augmented reality. The creation of a 3D collaborative environment was possible using the head mounted displays and superimposing digital data on the real world (Schmalsteig et al., 1996).

AR can be applied for learning, entertainment, or edutainment by enhancing a user's perception of and interaction with the real world, in particular to enhance collaborative learning experiences (Billinghurst et al., 2001).

During the last decade, augmented reality helped to create innovative and interactive teaching methods which facilitate and acquisition and student discussion (Wu et al., 2013, Chen & Wang, 2015, Avila-Garzon et al., 2021).

AR can also support the teaching of natural science, as described by Shen et al. (2019). This technology assists learners in understanding the composition and the characteristics of matter, for example in the DNA double structure (as shown in Figure 6).

A lot of studies show that the application of AR technology can help to establish a link between virtual and real-world information for students. In particular in architectural and civil engineering (ACE), where AR possesses immense application potential (Diao & Shih, 2019, Albahbah, Kıvrak, & Arslan, 2021).

Other interesting application of AR in educational field is to teach academic skills to students with autism spectrum disorder (ASD) and intellectual and developmental disabilities (IDD) (Yakubova et al., 2021).

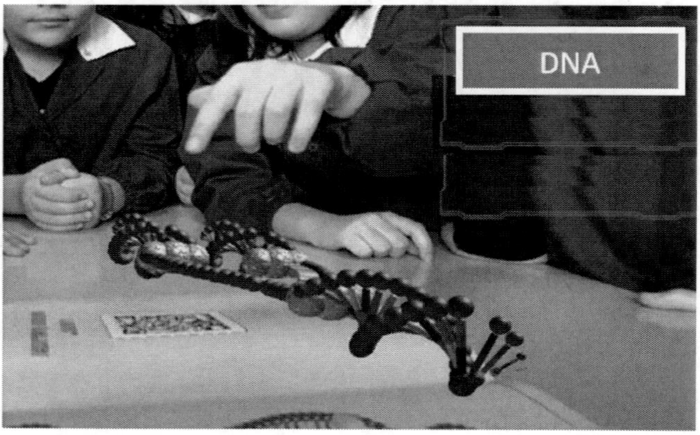

Figure 6. Augmented reality at primary school to discover the DNA double helix.

Several studies have applied various AR applications across different learning disciplines (Moro et al., 2021, Christopoulos et al., 2022; Mazzuco et al., 2022).

The advantage with the use of AR is mainly in the fact that there are no "real" errors in the learning situation. For example, if a surgeon learns laparoscopic surgery in a situation of augmented reality, there are no real consequences if errors are committed during exercise. Vice versa, this type of training offers the opportunity for more authentic learning and it permits the use of multiple learning styles.

4. Mixed Reality

Mixed reality can be considered as the merging of real and virtual worlds to produce new scenarios and new environments, where physical and digital objects can co-exist and interact together in real time (Croatti & Ricci, 2018). The term "mixed reality" was introduced in 1994 by Paul Milgram and Fumio Kishino in a work titled "A Taxonomy of mixed reality Visual Displays." They introduced Mixed Reality (MR), sometimes referred to as hybrid reality. They also described the "virtuality continuum" which extends itself from the completely real to the completely virtual environment passing through AR and augmented virtuality ranges. MR sometimes referred to as hybrid reality.

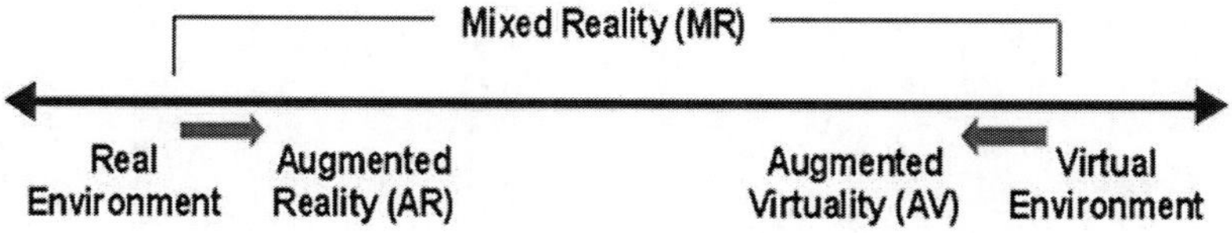

Figure 7. Reality-virtuality continuum (Milgram & Kishino, 1994).

Figure 7 shows the reality-virtuality continuum by Milgram and Kishino (1994), where is one part of the general area of mixed reality (van Krevelen & Poelman, 2010). In particular, they affirm that in virtual environments, VR can replace the surrounding environment by a virtual one. Figure 8 represents the interactions between computers, humans, and environments.

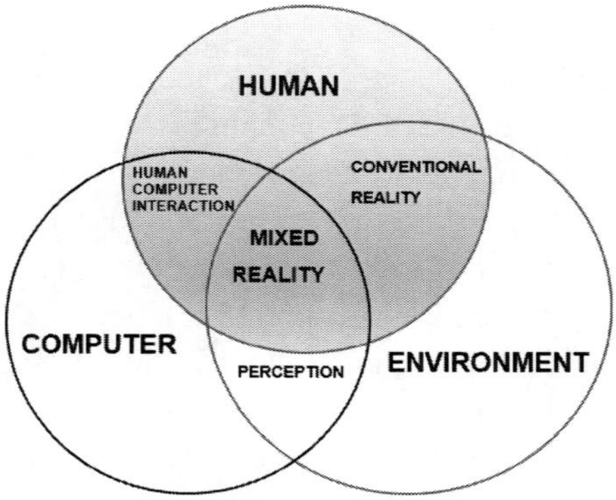

Figure 8. The interactions between computers, humans, and environments.

In 1994, Milgram and Kishimo described the hardware components for MR. They are:

- Monitor based (non-immersive) video displays, for example "window-on-the-world" (WoW) displays;
- Video displays that uses immersive head-mounted displays (HMD's);
- HMD's equipped with a see-through capability, with which computer generated graphics can be optically superimposed, using half-silvered mirrors, onto directly viewed real-world scenes;

- Same as the previous point, but using video, rather than optical, viewing of the "outside" world;
- Completely graphic display environments, either completely immersive, partially immersive or otherwise, to which video "reality" is added; and
- Completely graphic but partially immersive environments (e.g., large screen displays) in which real physical objects in the user's environment play a role in the computer generated scene, such as in reaching in and "grabbing" something with one's own hand.

MR has different application fields, in particular in education.

In 2005, Hughes et al. described how a multi-disciplinary research team transformed core MR technology and methods into diverse urban terrain applications. The applications described in their work are used for military training and situational awareness, as well as for community learning to significantly increase the entertainment, educational, and satisfaction levels of existing experiences in public venues.

Three years later, Callaghan et al. described a collaborative research, that involved three continents, towards creating "MiRTLE" a "mixed reality teaching & learning environment." This environment permitted to the teachers and students to participate in real time to mixed and online classes, interacting with avatar representations of each other (Callaghan et al., 2008). They also investigated how avatar representations of teachers and students helped to create a sense of shared presence, a sense of community and improving student engagement in online lessons.

Quint, Sebastian and Gorecki proposed, in 2015, a system architecture for a mixed-reality based learning environment. It combines physical objects and visualization of its digital content via Augmented Reality (Quint, Sebastian & Gorecki, 2015). In this research, MR is integrated with AR.

Dieker et al. (2016) describe the TeachLive™ Lab at the University of Central Florida (UCF) which is one of the first laboratories which uses a mixed reality simulation environment to prepare pre-service teachers or retrain in-service teachers. Tang et al. (2018) described a MR application for teaching product design to university students. They affirm that for students or individuals with learning difficulties, mixed reality allows interaction and feedback from the users. This aspect is particularly important for enhancing experience in teaching and learning. Moreover, the benefits to insert mixed reality into educational paths include better engagement, giving to the students the opportunities to experience and better remember what they have learned (Hughes et al., 2005).

VIRTUAL REALITY	AUGMENTED REALITY	MIXED REALITY
The user is immersed in a digital experience, creating a digital simulation of a real environment. The real world is hidden.	AR overlays digital information onto a real world. Interactive objects are layered on top of a physical environment without the ability to manipulate the augmented objects.	The capabilities of VR and AR are blended producing an environment where physical and digital objects coexist and interact in real time.

Figure 9. Differences between VR, AR, and MR (Sala, 2021).

Yamazaki et al. (2021) explore the use of patient-specific virtual reality (VR) and mixed reality (MR) temporal bone models in anatomical teaching, pre-operative surgical planning and intra-operative surgical referencing. In this research, most participants are favorable about the VR model and considered head mounted display as superior to a flat computer screen, because it permits a good degree of immersion in the virtual environment.

5. VR, AR, and MR: Differences

There are differences between VR, AR, and MR. In particular, VR involves digital environment with a cut from the physical environment. AR involves environment with the addition of digital elements. MR involves a mix of aspect from both virtual and real environments with the involvements with digital elements. Figure 9 resumes the differences between these three technologies (Sala, 2021).

More recently, the term XR can be used to refer to VR, AR and MR technologies. Ziker, Truman, & Dodds (2021) refer on XR using the term "cross reality" instead of "extended reality." They affirm: "Cross Reality (XR) refers to a group of emerging technologies such as virtual reality (VR), augmented reality (AR), and virtual worlds (VWs) that involve the use of 3D models/simulations across physical, virtual, and immersive platforms. The path to optimizing the use of XR in education is not always easy to navigate" (Ziker, Truman, & Dodds, 2021, p. 55).

Flinn (2019) defines XR as "the umbrella encompassing the virtual experience design space; that is all of MR (including AR and AV) and VR experiences." Figure 10, adapted from Flinn (2019), and Figure 11 offer two representations how AR, VR, MR, and XR are organized.

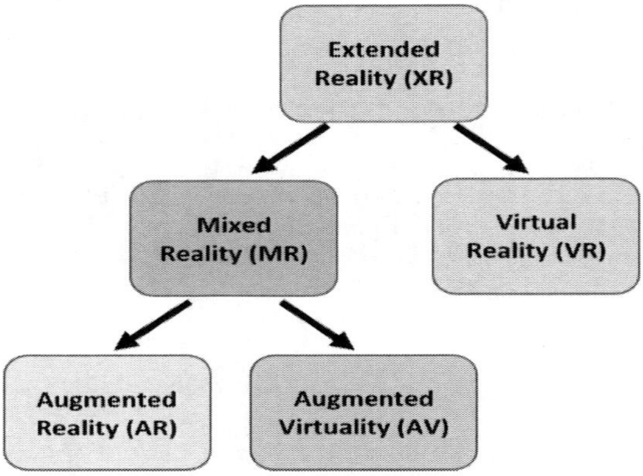

Figure 10. Representation how AR, VR, MR, and XR are organized, adapted from Flinn (2019).

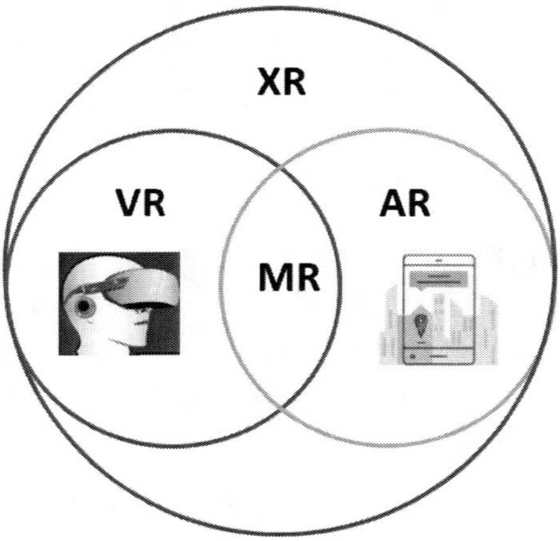

Figure 11. Organization of XR technology.

6. Future Trends

The unexpected breakout of Covid 19, induced by a Corona Virus (SARS-CoV-2), terrified the world. School and education are two of the notable sectors that are affected. During the pandemic, tools like remote meeting applications, online exams, VR, AR, MR were used to improve the quality of education (Raja & Lakshmi Priya, 2022).

Technological evolution, forced by pandemic, will open new scenarios and applications of XR. Recent studies that involve XR technology describe how they can support science, technology, engineering, the arts and mathematics (STEAM) learning (Ibáñez & Delgado-Kloos, 2018, Westlake, 2019, Wang, Ryoo, & Winkelmann, 2020, Kosko, Ferdig, & Roche, 2021, Xi, & Hamari 2021, Mystakidis, 2022).

In recent years, VR, AR, and MR have begun to take advantage of the wireless networks, but the problems connected to the bandwidth and the latency have limited the telepresence and collaborative virtual and augmented reality applications (Orlosky et al., 2017). New 5th generation mobile network can help to solve these problems. This technology is opening new scenarios in XR applications. 5G will reinvent digital media, by enabling us to step into a high-resolution 3D world, where the user will experience a new sense of immersion. It's possible to imagine a future where a surgeon, through a robotic interface, can reliably operate on patients in other isolated parts of the world (Kim et al., 2018).

Conclusion

This work describes a brief overview of the application of extended reality (VR, AR, and MR) in teaching and in learning environments. VR, AR and MR can interact and this hybridization suggests the introduction of a new term "extended reality" or "cross reality" (XR).

The application of these technologies in education can be seen as a set which influence, support and improve teaching methods, strengthening the educational process and helping to develop new ways of learning. Using XR technology the students can design their virtual world learning environments (Jacka & Booth, 2019).

There are still many problems to solve for the correct integration of XR technology in the schools.

In fact, in the fields of these technologies currently do not have universal standards that enable interoperability and seamless integration into existing software. It will be necessary the creation of norms and standards for implementing technologies in educational settings (Ziker, Truman, & Dodds, 2021). This will help to accelerate their adoption by educational institutions, but XR is not a panacea. It is a tool that blends the physical and digital, in particular ways and only its correct use can help to improve the teaching and learning paths.

References

Albahbah, M., Kıvrak, S., & Arslan, G. (2021). Application areas of augmented reality and virtual reality in construction project management: A scoping review. *Journal of Construction Engineering*, 4(3), 151-172.

Avila-Garzon, C., Bacca-Acosta, J., Duarte, J., & Betancourt, J. (2021). Augmented Reality in Education: An Overview of Twenty-Five Years of Research. *Contemporary Educational Technology*, 13(3).

Bhattarai, A., Alsadoon, A., Prasad, P. W. C., Pham, L., Haddad, S., Hsu, J., & Deva, A. (2019). A novel multiple communication paths for surgical telepresence videos delivery of the maxilla area in oral and maxillofacial surgery. *International Journal of Computer Assisted Radiology and Surgery*, 14(5), 873-883. doi:10.100711548-018-01904-y PMID:30649669.

Billinghurst, M., Kato, H., & Poupyrev, I. (2001). The MagicBook: A transitional AR interface. *Computers & Graphics*, 25(5), 745-753. doi:10.1016/S0097-8493(01) 00117-0.

Byrne, C. M. (1996). *Water on tap: The use of virtual reality as an educational tool* (Doctoral dissertation). University of Washington.

Callaghan, V., Gardner, M., Horan, B., Scott, J., Shen, L., & Wang, M. (2008, August). A mixed reality teaching and learning environment. In *International Conference on Hybrid Learning and Education* (pp. 54-65). Springer, Berlin, Heidelberg.

Chen, C. P., & Wang, C. H. (2015, December). The effects of learning style on mobile augmented-reality-facilitated English vocabulary learning. In *2015 2nd International Conference on Information Science and Security (ICISS)* (pp. 1-4). IEEE. 10.1109/ ICISSEC.2015.7371036.

Christopoulos, A., Pellas, N., Kurczaba, J., & Macredie, R. (2022). The effects of augmented reality-supported instruction in tertiary-level medical education. *British Journal of Educational Technology*, 53(2), 307-325.

Croatti, A., & Ricci, A. (2018, June). A model and platform for building agent-based pervasive mixed reality systems. In *International Conference on Practical Applications of Agents and Multi-Agent Systems* (pp. 127-139). Springer. 10.1007/978-3-319-94580-4_10.

Diao, P. H., & Shih, N. J. (2019). Trends and research issues of augmented reality studies in architectural and civil engineering education - A review of academic journal publications. *Applied Sciences*, 9(9), 1840.

Flinn, D. (2019). *VR...AR...MR...XR? WTFR They?* Retrieved 8th January 2022 https://medium.com/desn325-emergentdesign/vr-ar-mr-xr-wtfr-they-ce077312268a.

Garb, Y. (Winter 1987). Virtual Reality, *Whole Earth Review,* (57).

Ghezzi, T. L., & Corleta, O. C. (2016). 30 years of robotic surgery. *World Journal of Surgery*, 40(10), 2550-2557. doi:10.100700268-016-3543-9 PMID:27177648.

Guérin, E., Tosan, E., & Baskurt, A. (2002). Modeling and approximation of fractal surfaces with projected IFS attractors. In *Emergent Nature: Patterns, Growth and Scaling in the Science*. World Scientific.

Heilbrun, A., & Stacks B. (1989). Virtual reality. An Interview with Jaron Lanier. *Whole Earth Review*, 64, 108-119. Retrieved, 27 January 2022: http://www.jaronlanier.com/jaron%20whole%20earth%20review.pdf.

Höllerer, T. H., & Feiner, S. K. (2004). Mobile Augmented Reality. In H. A. Karimi & A. Hammad (Eds.), *Telegeoinformatics: Location-Based Computing and Services* (pp. 392-421). CRC Press.

Hosch, W. L. (2021). Augmented reality. *Encyclopedia Britannica*. Retrieved 20 January 2022, https://www.britannica.com/technology/augmented-reality.

Hughes, C. E., Stapleton, C. B., Hughes, D. E., & Smith, E. M. (2005). Mixed reality in education, entertainment, and training. *IEEE computer graphics and applications*, 25(6), 24-30.

Hurrell, C., & Baker, J. (2021). Immersive learning: Applications of virtual reality for undergraduate education. *College & Undergraduate Libraries*, 27(2-4), 197-209.

Ibáñez, M. B., & Delgado-Kloos, C. (2018). Augmented reality for STEM learning: A systematic review. *Computers & Education*, 123, 109-123. doi:10.1016/j.compedu.2018.05.002.

Jacka, L., & Booth, K. (2019). Students as designers of virtual world learning environments. In *Pre-Service and In-Service Teacher Education: Concepts, Methodologies, Tools, and Applications* (pp. 1697-1712). IGI Global. doi:10.4018/978-1-5225-7305-0.ch079.

Jin, M. L. E., Brown, M. M., Patwa, D., Nirmalan, A., & Edwards, P. A. (2021). Telemedicine, telementoring, and telesurgery for surgical practices. *Current problems in surgery*, 58(12), 100986.

Kim, S. S., Dohler, M., & Dasgupta, P. (2018). The Internet of Skills: Use of fifth-generation telecommunications, haptics and artificial intelligence in robotic surgery. *BJU International*, 122(3), 356-358. doi:10.1111/bju.14388 PMID:29750403.

Kosko, K. W., Ferdig, R. E., & Roche, L. (2021). Conceptualizing a shared definition and future directions for extended reality (XR) in teacher education. *Journal of Technology and Teacher Education*, 29(3), 257-277.

Latifi, K., & Latifi, R. (2018). Telemedicine and Telepresence for Surgery and Trauma. *Surgical Critical Care and Emergency Surgery: Clinical Questions and Answers*, 477-481.

Lowood, H. E (2021). Virtual reality. *Encyclopedia Britannica Retrieved 17 January 2022*, https://www.britannica.com/technology/virtual-reality.

Malik, C. A. J., & Hadi, S. (2021, November). The Design of Mini CNC Assembly Simulator Based on Virtual Reality Toolkit (VRTK). In *Journal of Physics: Conference Series* (Vol. 2111, No. 1, p. 012019). IOP Publishing.

Mazzuco, A., Krassmann, A. L., Reategui, E., & Gomes, R. S. (2022). A systematic review of augmented reality in chemistry education. *Review of Education*, 10(1), e3325.

Medium.com (2018). *What really is the difference between AR/MR/VR/XR?*. Retrieved 7th March 2022 https://medium.com/@northof41/what-really-is-the-difference-between-ar-mr-vr-xr-35bed1da1a4e.

Milgram, P., & Kishino, F. (1994). A taxonomy of mixed reality visual displays. *IEICE Trans. Information and Systems. E (Norwalk, Conn.)*, 77-*D*(12), 1321-1329. http://etclab.mie.utoronto.ca/people/paul_dir/IEICE94/ieice.html.

Mystakidis, S. (2022). Metaverse. *Encyclopedia*, 2(1), 486-497.

Moro, C., Phelps, C., Redmond, P., & Stromberga, Z. (2021). HoloLens and mobile augmented reality in medical and health science education: A randomised controlled trial. *British Journal of Educational Technology*, 52(2), 680-694.

Orlosky, J., Kiyokawa, K., & Takemura, H. (2017). Virtual and augmented reality on the 5G highway. *Journal of Information Processing*, 25(0), 133-141. doi:10.2197/ipsjjip. 25.133.

Pestalozzi, H. (1803). *ABC der Anschauung, oder Anschauungs-Lehre der Massverhaltnisse* [*ABC of view, or view doctrine of mass relations*]. Gessner.

Quint, F., Sebastian, K., & Gorecky, D. (2015). A mixed-reality learning environment. *Procedia Computer Science*, 75, 43-48. doi:10.1016/j.procs.2015.12.199.

Raja M., & Lakshmi Priya, G.G. (2022). Using Virtual Reality and Augmented Reality with ICT Tools for Enhancing Quality in the Changing Academic Environment in COVID-19 Pandemic: An Empirical Study. In: Hamdan A., Hassanien A. E., Mescon T., Alareeni B. (eds) Technologies, Artificial Intelligence and the Future of Learning Post-COVID-19. *Studies in Computational Intelligence*, vol 1019. Springer, Cham. https://doi.org/10.1007/978-3-030-93921-2_26.

Riva, G. (2006). *Virtual reality.* In *Encyclopaedia of Biomedical Engineering*. John Wiley & Sons.

Rosenblum, L. J., & Cross, R. A. (1997). The challenge of virtual reality. In W. R. Earnshaw, J. Vince, & H. Jones (Eds.), *Visualization & Modeling* (pp. 325-399). Academic Press.

Sala, N. (2008). Fractal Geometry in Computer Science. In Orsucci F., Sala N. (eds), *Reflexing Interfaces: The Complex Coevolution of Information Technology Ecosystems*, Information Science Reference, IGI Global, Hershey, New York, pp. 308-328.

Sala, N. (2009). Fractal Geometry in Artificial Worlds and in Second Life. *Chaos and Complexity Letters*, 4(1), 23-34.

Sala, N. (2016). Virtual Reality and Education: Overview across Different Disciplines. In *Emerging Tools and Applications of Virtual Reality in Education* (pp. 1-25). IGI Global, Hershey.

Sala, N. (2021). Virtual reality, augmented reality, and mixed reality in education: A brief overview. In *Current and prospective applications of virtual reality in higher education* (48-73). IGI Global, Hershey.

Sala, N., Metzeltin, S., & Sala, M. (2002). Applications of mathematics in the real world: territory and landscape. *Proceedings International Conference the Humanistic Renaissance in Mathematics Education*, 326-333.

Sala, N., & Sala, M. (2005). Virtual reality in education. In D. Carbonara (Ed.), *Technology literacy applications in learning environments* (pp. 358-367). Idea Group Inc. doi:10. 4018/978-1-59140-479-8.ch025.

Schmalsteig, D., Fuhrmann, A., Szalavari, Z., & Gervautz, M. (1996). Studierstube - An Environment for Collaboration in Augmented Reality. *CAVE '96 Workshop Proceedings.'*

Shakya, K., Khanal, S., Alsadoon, A., Prasad, P. W. C., Hsu, J., Deva, A., Elchouemic, A. (2019). Remote surgeon hand motion and occlusion removal in mixed reality in breast surgical telepresence: Rural and remote care. *American Journal of Applied Sciences*, 15(11), 497-509. doi:10.3844/ajassp.2018.497.509.

Shen, L. C., Wu, T. T., & Hsu, W. C. (2019, December). The Application of Augmented Reality to the Education of Chemistry - Take the Course of Nature Science in Junior High School as an Example. In *International Conference on Innovative Technologies and Learning* (pp. 41-48). Springer. 10.1007/978-3-030-35343-8_5.

Tsai, J. P., Kao, Y. C., & Lee, R. S. (2012, July). Investigating the effect of virtual reality application on teaching assistance for machine tools operation education. In *2012 IEEE/ASME International Conference on Advanced Intelligent Mechatronics (AIM)* (pp. 626-631). IEEE. 10.1109/AIM.2012.6265919.

van Krevelen, D. W. F., & Poelman, R. (2010). A survey of augmented reality technologies, applications and limitations. *The International Journal of Virtual Reality: a Multimedia Publication for Professionals*, 9(2), 1-20. doi:10.20870/IJVR.2010.9.2.2767.

Wang, M., Ryoo, J., & Winkelmann, K. (2020). Preface to the special issue on Cross Reality (XR) and Immersive Learning Environments (ILE) in education. *Interactive Learning Environments*, 28(5), 539-542.

Westlake, J. (2019). Exploring the Potential of Using Augmented Reality and Virtual Reality for STEM Education. In *Learning Technology for Education Challenges: 8th International Workshop, LTEC 2019*, Proceedings (36-44). Springer.

Whyte, J. (2002). *Virtual Reality and the Built Environment,* Architectural Press, Oxford.

Winn, W. (1993). *A conceptual basis for educational applications of virtual reality (Technical Report TR-93-9)*. Human Interface Technology Laboratory, University of Washington. Retrieved from http://www.hitl.washington.edu/publications/r-93-9/.

Wu, P. H., Hwang, G. J., Yang, M. L., & Chen, C. H. (2018). Impacts of integrating the repertory grid into an augmented reality-based learning design on students' learning achievements, cognitive load and degree of satisfaction. *Interactive Learning Environments*, 26(2), 221-234. doi:10.1080/10494820.2017.1294608.

Xia, S. B., & Lu, Q. S. (2021). Development status of telesurgery robotic system. *Chinese Journal of Traumatology*, 24(03), 144-147.

Xi, N., & Hamari, J. (2021). Shopping in virtual reality: A literature review and future agenda. *Journal of Business Research*, 134, 37-58.

Yakubova, G., Defayette, M. A., Chen, B. B. et al. The Use of Augmented Reality Interventions to Provide Academic Instruction for Children with Autism, Intellectual, and Developmental Disabilities: an Evidence-Based Systematic Review. *Rev. J. Autism Dev. Disord.* (2021). https://doi.org/10.1007/s40489-021-00287-2.

Yamazaki, A., Ito, T., Sugimoto, M., Yoshida, S., Honda, K., Kawashima, Y., & Tsutsumi, T. (2021). Patient-specific virtual and mixed reality for immersive, experiential anatomy education and for surgical planning in temporal bone surgery. *Auris Nasus Larynx*, 48(6), 1081-1091.

Ziker, C., Truman, B., & Dodds, H. (2021). Cross reality (XR): Challenges and opportunities across the spectrum. *Innovative learning environments in STEM higher education: Opportunities, challenges, and looking forward*, 55-77.

Chapter 10

Educational Robotics in Learning Paths

Raimondo Sgrò[*]
Elettra Robotics Lab, Lecco LC, Italy

Abstract

Robotics is an engineering discipline that studies and develops methodological approaches that allow a robot to perform specific tasks by automatically reproducing human work. This work aims to describe how robotics finds application in educational fields and in different learning paths.

Keywords: competition, cooperative learning, education, learning path, robotics, STEM

Introduction

The human being is at the top of the evolutionary chain. However, most of our behavior is deeply rooted in our history and results from the development of our species. In fact, we cannot affirm that the human being is a completely rational being: sometimes he/she manifests entirely irrational behavior, even his/her learning path can be full of practices that, although usual, are perfectly antithetical to rationality. How can robotics help us in learning paths? The answer is undoubtedly in the fascination that this exerts on young people, in the strategies that are adopted during the development of a didactic path and

[*] Corresponding Author's Email: info@elettraroboticslab.it.

In: Neuroscience and Technology Transform the Educational Ecosystem
Editors: Franco F. Orsucci and Nicoletta Sala
ISBN: 979-8-88697-157-6

how these adapt to the relational thinking model of the young homo sapiens. Not only do the possibilities of that individual depend on the success of the educational and training path, but also on the potential that the whole society can draw from its members, in the interest of common improvement and good. It is not, in fact, from a certain degree of flattening that social improvement is achieved, but from how each individual is able to grow and realize himself/herself by reaching the maximum of his/her potential.

1. Learning Methods

In 1955, Professor Johan Huizinga stated in his *Homo Ludens*: "Play is older than culture" [1, p. 1]. This observation allows us to link the act of playing to the social evolution of the human being. The roots of the game actually lie in the animal world and are part of the origins of mankind. Its primary function is to transmit information or prepare for future behavior. In only one word: to instruct. The game represents the ancestral way in which animal species, including humans, pass information down to new generations. Since playing has always been a natural behavior strongly rooted in our history and genes, it exerts a great charm on us. Evolution is necessarily based on effective mechanisms, so this practice is reliable and should not be boring or affected by other problems, which we can define as more modern. During its evolution, however, in parallel with language, man necessarily had to develop a method of transmitting information that conveyed a greater amount of data. Therefore, frontal teaching has become more prominent. The two ways are often side by side. Let us think, for example, of the training of artists or artisans who used to work "in the workshop." Today we would define this method by using the terms *coaching, apprenticeship* or even *learning by doing*. The Japanese culture provides a formidable example in this regard: traditionally knowledge is more 'stolen' by the learner who observes the teacher, rather than actively handed down [2]. Frontal transmission, although much more effective from the point of view of information flow, is however less rooted in our genes and affected by some collateral problems, such as being 'boring' to the learner. In order to understand this mechanism, we must acknowledge what rules it. Learning follows from the need for knowledge, useful knowledge that allows you to survive. For example, the necessity to respond to a need or, in other words, a motivation [3]. To be motivated, therefore, the individual must realize that he/she has such a need. If the social motivations fail, as it seems the case in the Western world today, the mechanism will break down. Learning will be perceived as useless, and the school, which is the main place of learning, will suffer the same fate.

What is the game based on? On the simulation of specific behavior or projection of reality. In the ancestral idea such behavior should have been useful in life. The lioness teaches her cubs to hunt, as well as children still play war: an activity that has unfortunately been characterizing our evolution for a long time. These elements have always triggered the imagination of young people. A fitting example is that of the phenomenon of online games, which only operate in a reality directed by rules of its own. Unfortunately, this activity can end up, in extreme cases, occupying many hours of real life, forming an additional problem. Therefore, young people are willing to spend time and energy in activities that involve projections of reality, because this behavior is perceived as natural. Another important problem in frontal learning concerns the generational gap between teacher and learner. In fact, the teacher may be perceived as a distant figure instead of being seen as social reference model (but this is another problem). The serious thing, actually, is that it often happens that the teacher is not listened to when he/she tries to put the learner in front of social problems. This is because, from the students' point of view, what the teacher says appear completely theoretical and unrelated to direct experience. In playful learning, there is an immediate action-reaction response. If there is also the element of competition in the game, and as a rule it is, it all looks even more appealing. Competitive behavior or the formation of groups with specific objectives are also ancestral for man and as such innate. It is no coincidence that in some companies, role-playing games or team sports are practiced as team building activities.

Obviously, frontal learning is indispensable due to its great ability to transmit information: not everything can be experienced directly. In fact, the human being also needs to learn to operate with abstract concepts. Nevertheless, frontal teaching is not the only tool available. Robotics competitions are a great environment on which to employ learning through play.

2. Students and Their Motivation

For those involved in teaching, or for anyone who is in contact with student generations, it is now evident that there is a progressive decrease in students' motivation. In fact, we have moved from a society in which schooling was a social goal to be achieved, to one in which this intrinsic value of education appears to be less and less strong [3]. This problem is widespread throughout the Western world, although some countries face it more successfully - the OECD-PISA results [5], provide us with data to reflect on. Of course, these results relate to learning and not directly to motivation, but there is a close correlation between the two. From a first reading it would seem that the link between favorable social conditions and academic success is rather complex, in fact many factors come into play in the latter with a rather difficult balance. Accordingly, the results concerning mathematical subjects are quite representative: the best results are achieved by students from four Chinese provinces.

As we said, the human being does not always have completely rational behavior. This is even more true in the period of formation and, specifically, during adolescence when the young must gain experience for their own growth and the construction of their own personality. In that time, the perception of one's own future appears as quite distant: adolescents do not have a clear idea of the link with future implications and, if on the one hand, growing within a system made of soft rules favors the development of individuality, on the other hand the risks of falling into one of the many traps that the path offers are high. For example, the filter of the medias (and even more so of social media) has a very strong impact on the young person. Conversely, a more rigid system of rules ensures better average results but often compresses individualities. Not all countries face this problem in the same way because, indeed, there are very different visions of the world. We may prefer a soft system but this must be carefully balanced with greater attention with the individual growth of the person and his/her learning styles [7]. As a consequence, an ineffective training and growing path has a significant impact on the future of the person. In fact, we can affirm that the unmotivated student will become unmotivated worker since the lack of motivation does not only concern the student but also the person and therefore will accompany him/her during the path of personal and professional growth. The picture that emerges is certainly alarming, because the world economic system is highly competitive and those who compete for the market do so thanks to a high level of knowledge and innovation, but all this requires passion and dedication. Just to dispel any doubt, all this does not mean that today's students are worse (or better) than the past ones, but simply that the social context in which they grow leads them to live a saturation of the senses behind standardizing models, and to develop motives certainly weaker than their peers who grew up in other contexts.

One can of course argue a lot about this issue. What is certain is that there are no easy remedies for this problem. Today, this is the main challenge that every teacher faces every time he/she enters the classroom and prepares to teach. It is a challenge that would need proper social recognition, but this topic is beyond our discussion. The point is, it is not possible to solve motivational problems upstream, this would require a synergistic action that the school alone is not able to implement. However, we must not be discouraged, since we can (and must) consider motivation as a didactic element, as part of the training and educational path, not as an independent element, stable in time, but as a factor to be stimulated and monitored. Motivation is therefore an element to be built. This goal can be achieved, for example, by carrying out activities that involve the class, or by creating a pleasant learning experience [3]. Robotics has the great advantage of involving students and even engaging them, so it is a very important motivational tool. Motivation is, in fact, the first step towards achieving positive learning outcomes, so that the virtuous circle is triggered (Figure 1):

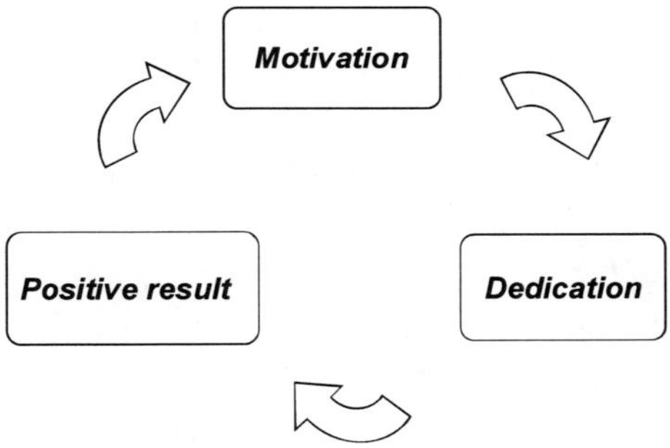

Figure 1. Representation of the virtuous teaching circle, where motivation is reinforced by the achievement of positive results.

3. Group Dynamics

Group dynamics have governed our species since the beginning of time thus generating instincts and behavior that we still carry with us. Living beings are moved by two main instincts: species conservation and individual conservation, and in this the human being is no exception. Most of our behavior has been shaped on these basic instincts. The organization in social agglomerations leads on one hand to optimize the chances of survival but on the other it creates a field of continuous confrontation between individuals. If sublimated, these instincts lead to mechanisms of virtuous growth, but this is not always the case. All this leads to the fact that the young man is driven on the one hand by the desire for aggregation and acceptance, on the other by the desire to emerge and excel within the group. Unfortunately, we may witness situations in which these types of behavior are extreme, thus leading in some cases to despicable phenomena such as bullying, However, these same practices can well governed and understood and, as a consequence, create for the young person an environment suitable for his/her growth. It is no coincidence that in the OECD-PISA survey, there are indicators related to both collaboration and competition between students [6]. Group dynamics are essential for a socially healthy growth of the young person, establishing a safe context where the rules of comparison help its same creation. In this sense, robotic competitions offer an opportunity to achieve this type of goal. In fact, there is of course the work of the group, with a sharing of objectives, and also the aspect of competition. Both aspects must necessarily be virtuous, and the role of the teacher, who works in that *mentoring* context, is indispensable to guide young people towards virtuous attitudes.

3.1. Group Work as a Learning Tool

In the strategic plan for the 2020-2024 period, the European Union has given great value to learning paths in the digital age, not only promoting greater inclusiveness in the pathways but also specifically encouraging pathways related to STEM (Science, Technology, Engineering and Mathematics) and artificial intelligence [4]. It is certainly not easy to combine these elements, which represents additional challenge for teachers. Teaching, in fact, is not only the main tool on which the transmission of knowledge is based, but also offers opportunities to experiment and learn social and professional practices.

The methodology of cooperative learning and its advantages are well known [9, 10]. So, applying the tool of teamwork to educational robotics represents an opportunity to improve learning experience, which, if properly arranged, allows individual students to operate in resonance with the already discussed features of educational robotics [8].

In order to avoid any doubt, I would like to draw a clear definition of teamwork. It is well known that there may be some downsides to this practice. For example, negative school experiences of teamwork in which work is mainly carried out by one person, to be benefited by all members, with the consequence that there is no improvement in learning, since only one person has worked. Indeed, there is a deterioration compared to individual work. This creates a situation of frustration on the part of the student who has had to support the entire group with his work, resulting in a loss of confidence in the school system. Such experiences are known and should be kept in mind as models to be avoided. What should be done instead is to be inspired by the model of cooperative learning when the group works to achieve a goal for which the work of all the members is necessary. Interdependence and individual responsibility are fundamental requirements for success.

3.2. Structuring Groups: Interaction and Responsibility

A robotics project is certainly suitable for group management. In particular, this is even more evident in a Technical Secondary School, where the project can be articulated both on hardware and software. On the curricular level, it is important that the groups are homogeneous, in the sense that there should be no disadvantaged or otherwise unbalanced groups. Therefore, in supporting the spontaneous formation of working groups, the teacher must also prevent that the aforementioned imbalances do not arise, intervening where necessary. In this way, on the one hand, the cohesion of the group is fostered, on the other hand, by exploiting the existing social ties, o equal opportunities of learning are monitored. Within the group, clear responsibilities must be identified in accordance with the principles set out above.

For example, if the hardware is divided into blocks, each individual can take care of the realization of a block. It is also possible to operate a division between those who will deal with hardware and those of software, even if this division may be critical as it is likely to preclude part of the learning experience to some members of the group. The division of tasks must stimulate interactions. In fact, as the various blocks of the system must communicate with each other, the respective designers will have to exchange information, otherwise the project will not work. The interaction between the members of the group must represent a necessity rather than an imposition, a natural fact to which the group must adapt spontaneously. Interaction and exchange of information are indispensable elements for modern working life. In fact, it is not only necessary to be able to communicate correctly using a correct technical language, but also to establish social interactions of positive collaborations. In general, the experiences lived together improve the group bonds, so these types of formative activities help to fix such experiences and make them heritage for the students' growth.

The principle of individual responsibility is apparently in opposition to the concept of group work, but, as I have already pointed out, all those situations in which the group becomes a shield that hides those who do not work should be avoided. It is possible to identify clear responsibilities for each member of the team, indeed this is a crucial point. Responsibilities must be carefully chosen by the teacher since they should not be too uneven. It is also important not to create marked hierarchies that could disturb the process of learning and socialization. Each member of the group must be and feel responsible and necessary.

At this point, understanding how to ensure the homogeneity of learning experiences, together with avoiding differences or incomplete knowledge forced by the division of roles, become fundamental. The answer is quite simple: as in any working group, while maintaining their responsibilities, it is good that everyone has knowledge of the results achieved by others. This also avoids deadlocks, which would waste time in the absence of one of the members of the group. This point also needs to be made clear: in the final verification phase, each member of the group will also answer questions concerning the work done by the others. This encourages interaction.

The role of the mentor/teacher is fundamental in this type of path, because on the one hand it supervises the relationships within the group so that they always remain correct, on the other hand it establishes the objectives of the path, knows how to explain them to students so that they have a positive virtuous - model.

4. The Role of Robots in Learning

Robotics is a fascinating discipline, that's a fact. It captures students' interest. Where the secret of this charm lies is not easy to understand but it probably lies in the fact of providing the possibility to create an object that somehow emulates a living being that, to some extent, can be seen as an artificial alter-ego. Nonetheless, robotics is not a simple discipline. In fact, if faced superficially it can lead the young person to become discouraged.

The market is now full of kits for educational purpose that greatly facilitate the task of the teacher. However, if the goal is to obtain professional skills, the use of kits should be overcome. Robotics in its educational form offers the possibility of being used as a transversal means, either to motivate students or as a means of teaching specific knowledge, and sometimes both at the same time. The research of motivation by the student is often a delicate process, and the break of the virtuous circle between motivation and learning can lead to serious consequences, such as also abandoning school.

Let's see what kinds of learning an educational robotics project is suitable for. Clearly it is quite immediate to imagine learning paths related to the fundamental disciplines to which robotics is linked, namely electronics, computer science and mechanics, but other disciplines such as physics or mathematics may be also involved. Overall, it is easy to think about so-called STEM pathways. The teacher is therefore free to build paths that highlight only one of these aspects or more than one. Based on our experience, we believe that a complete design path of a robot is the most to aspire to both if you want to transmit specific professional technical knowledge, whether you want to tackle transversal skills such as project chain and *problem solving*. Indeed, there is also another aspect to be considered, the robot could be viewed as a mediator, which is often relied on, and in some cases facilitates relationships and learning even for those students who have problems in the relational sphere.

5. The Importance of Sharing in Education

If common goals are perceived as shared, the group works better. This aspect depends both on the perception of the individual but also on how the group itself knows how to adapt and relate to its members. In the growing paths, education to the contradictory is fundamental: it is important in our working and social life, it cannot be avoided, so it is worth trying to educate the young person to civil confrontation through the use of precise rules. As it is well known, learning is more effective if not only our brain but also our senses, interactions and emotions are involved. A positive experience leads to strengthening what has been learned, on the contrary a negative one tends to lead the student to forget what has already been learned. There are not only successful experiences in life, therefore it is important to prepare the young student to manage failure, too. Sometimes, even if the group has had a positive experience, it is not granted that all its members have had the same perception. Therefore, it is important to plan and implement moments in which students listen to each other, exchange and compare within the group so that all points of view can be made explicit.

While carrying out an educational project, such as educational robotics, it is very useful to gradually switch from the vertical model to the circular one (Figure 2). The latter, in fact, is not very widespread, because it often generates in the teacher the fear that the situation can somehow get out of hand. It is the author's opinion that this model should be the one to be aimed at, not only within the management of a project, but also for the organization of the school and society.

In learning and school life, as in working life, there are not only goal-oriented interactions, each group is a social agglomeration, so it also lives from other interactions whose existence should not be neglected. It is not always easy to explore the social dynamics of a group, many of them can be ignored by the teacher, in this regard it may be useful to create moments of sharing at the end of a fixed path. The author has been able to verify with several years of experience, the benefit that these moments have, often emerge not obvious aspects. It is very important to establish very clear rules, so that each element of the group has the same space and the same possibility to provide both a self-assessment, and to evaluate the work of the rest of the group, making both positive and negative criticisms (with the obvious rule not to offend anyone). It is important that the learner has his moment of free expression, and in this no one else must be able to intervene, not even the mentor, who will have to watch over compliance with the rules of sharing.

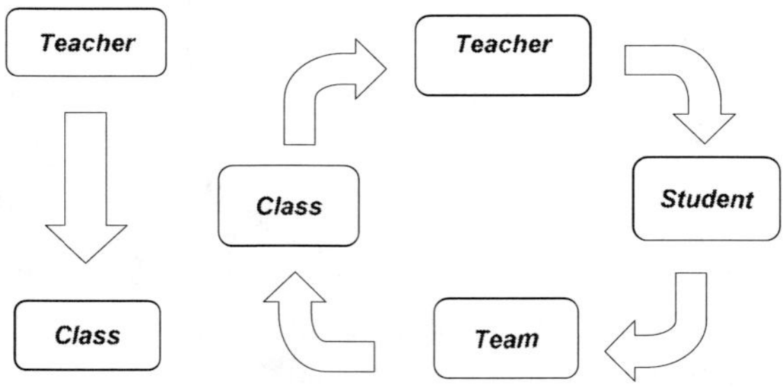

Figure 2. Representation of the teacher class relation: on the left the vertical process in the frontal teaching, on the right the circular link to be established in the collaborative project groups.

Only at the end, the teacher/mentor can draw conclusions from the experience, making a synthesis of the views expressed, without ever blaming the students but always trying to value the positive and constructive aspects, cementing ties, making sure that even from failure, students do not draw disappointment but examples to continue the activity. Students must be able to add even the smallest tool to their education, which may be the management of failure, a very useful tool in real life.

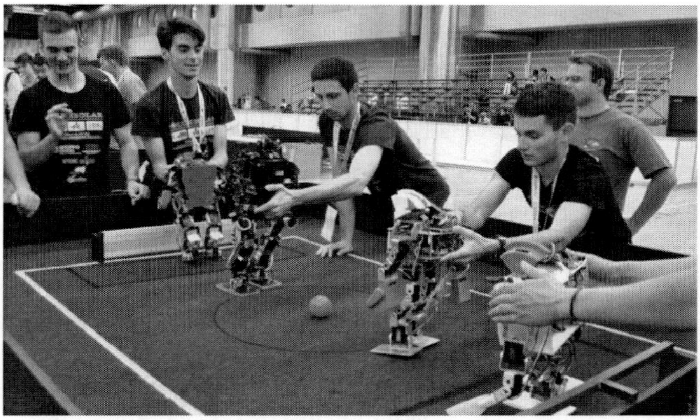

a)

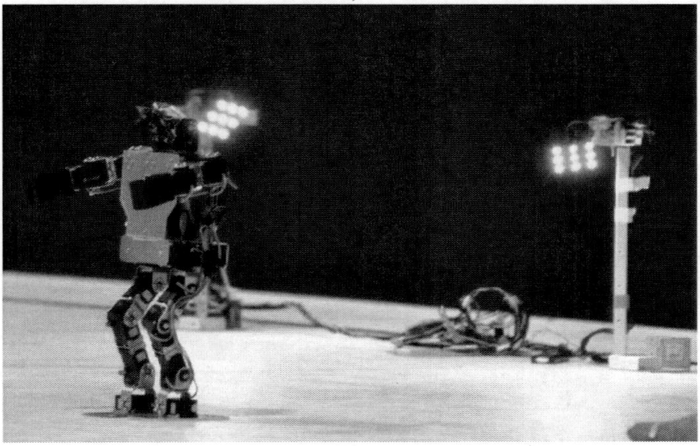

b)

Figure 3. Some moments takes from RoboCup Junior competitions (by courtesy of the author).

Conclusion

Robotics is widely applied in the educational field [11, 12, 13, 14]. The purpose of this work has been to describe how robotics can be integrated into teaching through different methodologies and strengthening cooperation activities.

I can therefore summarize some key elements that I have highlighted above:

- balance between playful learning and formal learning;
- motivations related to robotics in STEM pathways;
- group work, sharing of objectives and experiences.

It has been shown how it is possible to create paths of educational robotics that link these elements. Indeed, this is not the only possible method, but this is reinforced by many years of experience. In addition, there is another element that connects with the previous ones very well, namely competition.

The Figures 3a and 3b reproduce some moments takes from RoboCup Junior competitions.

From this deep analysis, it is possible to understand the extent to which this element is rooted in us and this offers us the possibility to realize educational paths set within robotic competitions, combining these four elements and, at the same time, strengthening them.

References

[1] Huizinga, J. (1955). *Homo Ludens: A Study of the Play-Element in Culture*, Paperback, London.

[2] Ratti, O, Westbrook, A. (1996). *I segreti dei samurai* [Secrets of the samurai], Mediterranee, Roma 1996.

[3] Gatti, R. (2002). *Saper sapere. La motivazione come obiettivo educativo* [*Knowing how to know Motivation as an educational objective*], Carrocci, Urbino.

[4] https://ec.europa.eu/info/system/files/eac_sp_2020_2024_en.pdf.

[5] OECD (2019), *PISA 2018 Results (Volume I): What Students Know and Can Do*, PISA, OECD Publishing, Paris, https://doi.org/10.1787/5f07c754-en.

[6] OECD (2019), *PISA 2018 Results (Volume III): What School Life Means for Students' Lives*, PISA, OECD Publishing, Paris, https://doi.org/10.1787/acd78851-en.

[7] Dunn, R., Learning styles: Theory, research, and practice. *National Forum of Applied Educational Research Journal*, 13.

[8] Sgrò, R. (2010) La robotica negli istituti tecnici industriali: tra motivazione giovanile, innovazione e realtà (acd) *Atti del Convegno ROBOSCUOLA 2010*, Vicenza 15 aprile 2010 [Robotics in industrial technical institutes: between youth motivation, innovation and reality (acd) *Proceedings of the ROBOSCUOLA 2010 Conference*, Vicenza 15 April 2010].

[9] Sharan, Y., Sharan, S. (1998). *Gli alunni fanno ricerca, l'apprendimento in gruppi cooperative* [*Pupils do research, learning in cooperative groups*], Erickson.

[10] Johnson, D. W., Johnson, R. T., & Smith, K. A. (2000). *Cooperative learning.* Minneapolis, MN, 88.

[11] Jung, S. E., & Won, E. S. (2018). Systematic review of research trends in robotics education for young children. *Sustainability*, 10(4), 905.
[12] Daniela, L., & Lytras, M. D. (2019). Educational robotics for inclusive education. *Technology, Knowledge and Learning*, 24(2), 219-225.
[13] López-Belmonte, J., Segura-Robles, A., Moreno-Guerrero, A. J., & Parra-González, M. E. (2021). Robotics in education: a scientific mapping of the literature in Web of Science. *Electronics*, 10(3), 291.
[14] Cobello, S., & Milli, E. (2022). Sociological Aspects of Educational Robotics. In *How World Events Are Changing Education* (pp. 150-158). Brill.

Chapter 11

Fractal Geometry in Computer Graphics and in Virtual Reality*

Nicoletta Sala†
Academy of Architecture, University of Italian Switzerland,
Largo Bernasconi, Mendrisio, Switzerland
Department of Informatics and Communication,
University of Insubria, Varese, Italy

Abstract

Fractal geometry is also known as "Mandelbrot's geometry" in honour to its "father" the mathematician Benoit Mandelbrot (b. 1924), that showed how fractals can occur in many different places in mathematics, in physics and in other disciplines.

Fractal geometry can be used for modelling natural shapes (e.g., fern, trees, seashells, rivers, mountains), and its important applications also appear in computer science, because this "new" geometry permits to compress the images, to reproduce, in the virtual reality environments, the complex patterns and the branching forms which are present in nature using simple iterative instructions. The aim of this paper is to present the applications of fractal geometry in computer graphics (to compress images) and in virtual reality (to generate virtual territories and landscapes).

---

* This article was originally published in Chaos and Complexity Letters, volume 3 number 2 (2009).

† Corresponding Author's Email: nsala@arch.unisi.ch.

In: Neuroscience and Technology Transform the Educational Ecosystem
Editors: Franco F. Orsucci and Nicoletta Sala
ISBN: 979-8-88697-157-6

Keywords: Fractal Geometry, Self-Similarity, Iterated Function Systems, L-Systems, Fractional Brownian Motion, Computer Graphics, Virtual Reality, Virtual World

1. Introduction

French mathematicians Pierre Fatou (1878-1929) and Gaston Julia (1893-1978) worked on fractals at the beginning of the 20th century. The word "Fractal" was coined by the Polish-born Franco-American Benoit Mandelbrot, and it derives from the Latin verb "frangere", "to break", and from the related adjective "fractus", "fragmented and irregular". This term denotes the geometry of nature, which traces inherent order in chaotic shapes and processes, and it was created to differentiate pure geometric figures from other types of figures that defy such simple classification. The Encyclopaedia Britannica introduces the fractal geometry as follow (2007): "In mathematics, the study of complex shapes with the property of self-similarity, known as fractals.

Rather like holograms that store the entire image in each part of the image, any part of a fractal can be repeatedly magnified, with each magnification resembling all or part of the original fractal. This phenomenon can be seen in objects like snowflakes and tree bark.... This new system of geometry has had a significant impact on such diverse fields as physical chemistry, physiology, and fluid mechanics; fractals can describe irregularly shaped objects or spatially nonuniform phenomena that cannot be described by Euclidean geometry".

The acceptance of the word "fractal" was dated in 1975, when Mandelbrot presented the list of publications between 1951 and 1975, date when the French version of his book was published, the people were surprised by the variety of the studied fields: Economy, linguistics, cosmology, noise on telephone lines, turbulence (Mandelbrot, 1975).

Mandelbrot's geometry replaces Euclidian geometry (which dominated our mathematical thinking for thousands of years) and it is recognized as the true geometry able to describe the Nature. Recently, the electronics evolution and the increase in the computer calculation power permitted connections between the fractal geometry and the other disciplines (for example, biology, economy, medicine, engineering, arts, architecture), and the multiplicity of applications had an important role in the diffusion of fractal geometry (Mandelbrot, 1982; Leland et al., 1993; Nonnenmacker et al., 1994; Eglash,

1999; Barnsley et al., 2002; Sala, 2006; Vyzantiadou et al., 2007). This paper is organized as follows: section 2 introduces the fractal objects, section 3 presents the application of the fractal geometry in computer graphics. Section 4 introduces the fractal geometry as a tool for modelling virtual landscapes. Section 5 is dedicated to the conclusions.

2. Fractal Objects

A fractal object could be defined as a fragmented geometric shape that can be subdivided in parts, each of which is approximately a reduced-size copy of the whole (Mandelbrot, 1982). Fractals are generally self-similar on multiple scales. So, all fractals have a built-in form of iteration or recursion. Sometimes the recursion is visible in how the fractal is constructed. For instance, the Koch snowflake, the Cantor set, and the Sierpinski triangle (figure 1a) are all generated using simple recursive rules. Self similarity is present in nature, too. Figures 1b shows a natural fractal object, the cauliflower which has the property of self similarity (it repeats its shape in different scales).

Different kinds of fractals (e.g., Iterated Function Systems and the Lindenmayer System) and the self similarity are applied in many fields of computer science, for example, in computer graphics, in virtual reality, and in the computer networks for controlling the traffic (Leland et al, 1992; Erramilli et al., 1993; Liu, 2006).

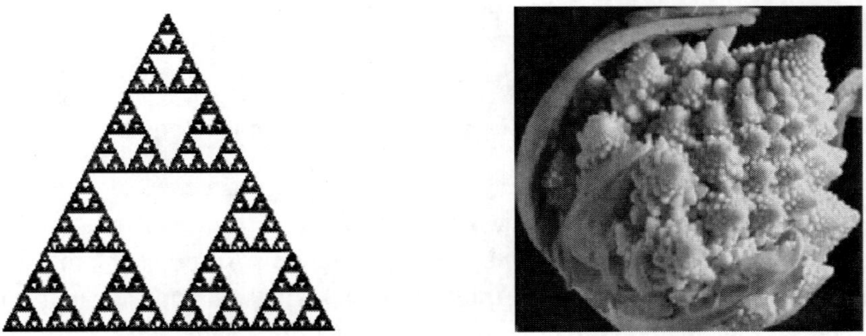

a) b)

Figure 1. a). The Sierpinski triangle is a fractal generated using simple geometric rules b).The cauliflower is a fractal present in the nature

2.1. The Self-Similarity

The invariance against changes in scale or size is named "self-similarity", and it is a property by which an object contains smaller copies of itself at arbitrary scales. Mandelbrot defined the self-similarity as follow: "When each piece of a shape is geometrically similar to the whole, both the shape and the cascade that generate it are called self-similar" (Mandelbrot, 1982, p. 34). "Similar" means that the relative proportions of the internal angles and shapes' sides remain the same. Mandelbrot (1982) observed that this property is ubiquitous in the natural world, and in the human body is possible to observe the presence of fractal geometry using two different points of view: temporal fractals and spatial fractals.

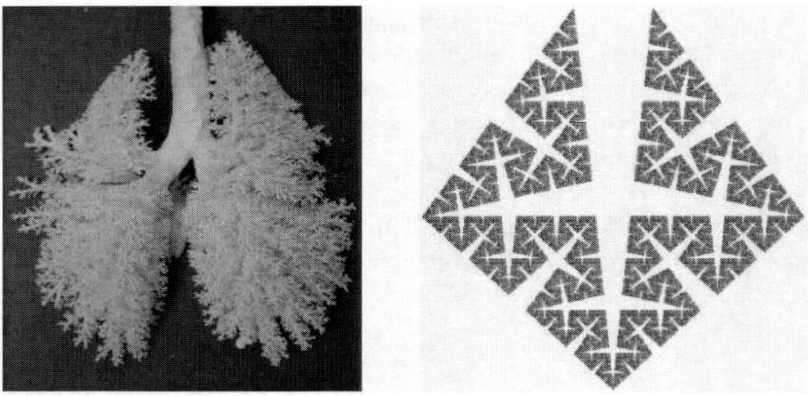

a) b)

Figure 2. Frontal view of dog's lungs a) it is a natural fractal object. "Fractal lungs" b) is a fractal generated using simple geometric rules, starting from two triangles.

Temporal fractals are present in some dynamic processes, for example in the cardiac rhythm. Spatial fractals refer to the presence of self-similarity observed to various enlargements, for instance, the small intestine repeats its form on different scales. Spatial fractals also refer to the branched patterns that are present inside the human body for enlarging the available surface for the absorption of the substances, and the distribution and the collection of the solutes occupying a relative small fraction of the body.

Figure 2a above shows the frontal view of dog's lungs. It is an example of self-similarity in the nature. In figures 2b there is an example of a fractal object which represents an attempt to reproduce complex shapes of the lungs, using few simple geometric rules.

2.2. The Iterated Function System

Iterated Function System (IFS) is another fractal that can be applied in computer science, in particular in computer graphics. Barnsley (1993, p. 80) defined the Iterated Function System as follow: “A (hyperbolic) iterated function system consists of a complete metric space (X, d) together with a finite set of contraction mappings w_n: X→ X with respective contractivity factor s_n, for n = 1, 2,.., N. The abbreviation “IFS” is used for “iterated function system”. The notation for the IFS just announced is {X, w_n, n = 1, 2,.., N} and its contractivity factor is $s = \max \{s_n : n = 1, 2, \ldots, N\}$.” Barnsley put the word “hyperbolic” in parentheses because it is sometimes dropped in practice. He also defined the following theorem (Barnsley, 1993, p. 81): “Let {X, w_n, n = 1, 2, … N} be a hyperbolic iterated function system with contractivity factor s. Then the transformation W: H(**X**) → H(**X**) defined by:

$$W(B) = \cup_{n=1}^{n} w_n(B) \tag{1}$$

For all B∈ H(X), is a contraction mapping on the complete metric space (H(X), h(d)) with contractivity factor s. That is:

$$H(W(B), W(C)) \leq s \cdot h(B,C) \tag{2}$$

for all B, C ∈ H(**X**). Its unique fixed point, A ∈ H(X), obeys

$$A = W(A) = \cup_{n=1}^{n} w_n(A) \tag{3}$$

and is given by $A = \lim_{n\to\infty} W^{on}(B)$ for any B ∈ H(X).”

The fixed point A ∈ H(X), described in the theorem by Barnsley is called the “attractor of the IFS” or “invariant set”.

Recall that an affine map of the plane is given by form:

$$w\begin{bmatrix}x\\y\end{bmatrix}=\begin{bmatrix}a & c\\b & d\end{bmatrix}\begin{bmatrix}x\\y\end{bmatrix}+\begin{bmatrix}e\\f\end{bmatrix}$$

and it is determined by six number, *a*, *b*, *c*, *d*, *e*, and *f*. The affine maps are combinations of translations, rotations and scalings in the plane. If the scaling factor is less than 1, we have contractive affine maps. In the case of IFS, Bogomolny (1998) affirms that two problems arise. One is to determine the fixed point of a given IFS, and it is solved by what is known as the "deterministic algorithm".

The second problem is the inverse of the first: for a given set A∈H(X), find an iterated function system that has A as its fixed point (Bogomolny, 1998). This is solved approximately by the Collage Theorem (Barnsley, 1993, p. 94).

The Collage Theorem states: "Let (X, d), be a complete metric space. Let L∈H(X) be given, and let ε ≥ o be given. Choose an IFS (or IFS with condensation) {X, (w_n), w_1, w_2,…, w_n} with contractivity factor 0 ≤ s ≤ 1, so that

$$h(L,\cup_{\substack{n=1\\(n=0)}}^{n} w_n(L)) \leq \varepsilon \tag{4}$$

where h(d) is the Hausdorff metric. Then

$$h(L,A) \leq \frac{\varepsilon}{1-s} \tag{5}$$

where A is the attractor of the IFS. Equivalently

$$h(L,A) \leq (1-s)^{-1} h(L,\cup_{\substack{n-1\\(n-0)}} w_n(L)) \tag{6}$$

for all L∈H(X)."

The Collage Theorem describes how to find an Iterated Function System whose attractor is "close to" a given set, one must endeavour to find a set of transformations such that the union, or collage, of the images of the given set under transformations is near to the given set.

2.3. L-Systems

Hungarian biologist Aristid Lindenmayer (1925-1989) introduced a kind of fractals, called L-systems, for modelling biological growth in 1968. L-system (or Lindenmayer system) is an algorithmic method for generating branched forms and structures such as plants. The components of an L-system are the following:

- An alphabet which is a finite set V of formal symbols containing elements that can be replaced (variables).
- the constants which is a set S of symbols containing elements that remain fixed.
- The axiom (also called the initiator) which is a string ω of symbols from V defining the initial state of the system.
- A production (or rewriting rule) P that is a set of rules or productions defining the way variables can be replaced with combinations of constants and other variables. A production consists of two strings - the predecessor and the successor.

The rules of the L-system grammar are applied iteratively starting from the initial state.

L-systems are also commonly known as "parametric L systems", and they are defined as a tuple $G = \{V, S, \omega, P\}$. L-system can be also defined as a formal grammar (a set of rules and symbols) most famously used for modelling the growth processes of plant development, and it has been thought able for modelling the morphology of a variety of organisms. Prusinkiewicz and Lindenmayer (1990) well described the differences between L-systems and Chomsky grammars. They affirmed: "The essential difference between Chomsky grammars and L-systems lies in the method of applying productions. In Chomsky grammars productions are applied sequentially, whereas in L-systems they are applied in parallel and simultaneously replace all letters in a given word. This difference highlights the biological motivation of L-systems. Productions are intended to capture cell divisions in multicellular organisms, where many divisions may occur at the same time. Parallel production application has an essential impact on the formal properties of rewriting systems" (Prusinkiewicz and Lindenmayer, 1990, pp. 2,3). Strings generated by L-systems may be interpreted geometrically in different ways. For instance, L-system strings serve a drawing commands for LOGO-style turtle.

Table 1. Commands for LOGO-style turtle derived by L-systems

Symbols	Meaning
F	Move forward a step of length s. The state of the turtle changes, now it is (x', y', α), where x' = x +s cos α and y'= y + s sin α. A segment between (x, y), starting point, and the point (x', y') is drawn.
f	Move forward a tep of length s without drawing a line.
+	Turn left by angle δ. The positive orientation of angles is counterclockwise, and the next state of the turtle is (x, y, α+δ).
-	Turn right by angle δ. The next state of the turtle is (x, y, α - δ).
[	Push the current state of the turtle onto a pushdown operations stack. The information saved on the stack contains the turtle's position and orientation, and possibly other attributes such as the color and width of lines being drawn.
]	Pop a state from the stack and make it the current state of the turtle. No line is drawn, although in general the position of the turtle changes.

Prusinkiewicz and Lindenmayer also defined a state of the turtle as a triplet (x, y, α), where the Cartesian coordinates (x, y) represent the turtle's position, and the angle α, called the heading, is interpreted as the direction in which the turtle is facing. Given the step size s and the angle increment δ, the turtle can respond to commands represented by the symbols in the table 1 above.

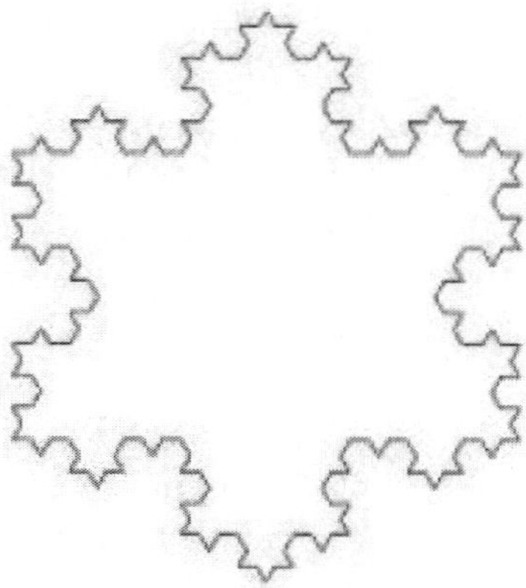

Figure 3. Koch snowflake generated by L-system.

The Koch snowflake can be simply encoded as a Lindenmayer system with initial string "F++F++F", string rewriting rule F → F-F++F-F, and angle 60°, as shown in figure 3.

3. Fractal Geometry in Computer Graphics

The computer graphics community has generalized the terms "fractal objects" outside Mandelbrot's original definition (Foley et al., 1997). It means anything that has a substantial measure of exact or statistical self-similarity. In the case of statistical fractals it is the probability density that repeats itself on every scale. An application of fractal geometry is in the compression of images (fractal compression). A fractal compression is performed by locating self-similar sections of an image, then using a fractal algorithm to generate the sections. A compressed image can be defined as follow: it is an encoding that describes (i) the grid partitioning, and (ii) the affine transformations (Shulman, 2000). Important researches on fractal image compression derived from the mathematical studies on chaos and fractals in the years 1978–1985, and Michael Barnsley was the principal researcher who worked on this. The basic idea was to represent by an Iterated Function System (IFS) of which the fixed point is close to that image (Barnsley, 1988; Barnsley et al., 1988). This fixed point is also known as "fractal" (Fisher, 1995). Each IFS is coded as a contractive transformation with coefficients. The Banach fixed point theorem (1922) guarantees the existence and uniqueness of fixed points of certain self maps of metric spaces, and provides a constructive method to find those fixed points.

An image can be represented using a set of IFS codes rather than pixels. Thus, a good compression ratio could be achieved. This method was good for generating almost real images based on simple iterative algorithms. The inverse problem, going from a given image to an Iterated Function System that can generate the original (or at least closely resemble it), was solved by Jacquin according to Barnsley in 1988. Jacquin introduced a modified scheme for representing images called Partitioned Iterated Function Systems (PIFS). The main characteristics of this approach were that (i) it relied on the assumption that image redundancy can be efficiently exploited through self-transformability on a block-wise basis, and (ii) it approximated an original image by a fractal image (Jacquin, 1992). In a PIFS, the transformations do not map from the whole image to the parts, but from larger parts to smaller parts. In the Jacquin's method, the small areas are called "range blocks", the big areas are called "domain blocks" and the pattern of range blocks was called the "partitioning of an image". Every pixel of the original image has to belong to one range block. This system of mappings is contractive, thus when iterated it quickly converge to its fixed point image. Thus, the key point for this algorithm is to find fractals which can best describe the original image and then to represent them as affine transformations.

All methods which are based on fractal transformations with Iterated Function Systems generate a close approximation of a scene using only few geometric transformations (Peitgen and Saupe, 1988; Wohlberg and de Jager, 1999; Zhao and Liu, 2005).

Fractal compression attempts to eliminate redundant or unnecessary information, and it is a lossy compression method (compressing data and then decompressing it retrieves data that may well be different from the original, but is close enough to be useful in some way). Most lossy compression formats suffer from generation loss: repeatedly compressing and decompressing the file will cause it to progressively lose quality (as shown in figure 4).

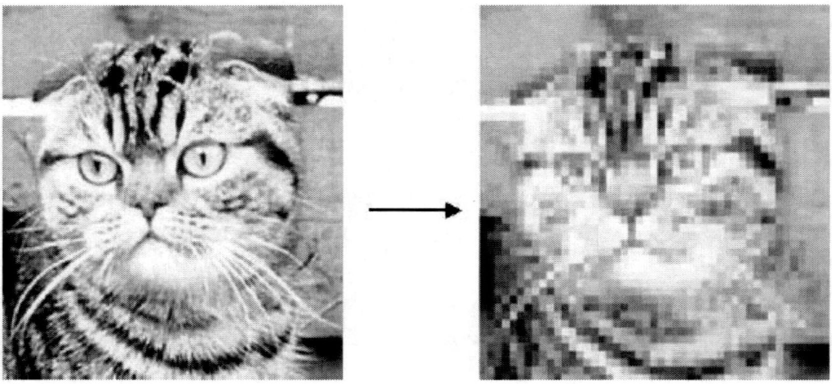

Figure 4. Fractal compression: repeatedly compressing and decompressing the file will cause it to progressively lose quality.

In the field of the compression of images new methods have been introduced. For example, van Wijk and Saupe (2004) present a fast method to generate fractal imagery based on Iterated Function Systems. The high performance derives from three factors: (i) all steps are expressed in graphics operations which can be performed quickly by hardware, (ii) frame to frame coherence is exploited, (iii) only a few commands per image have to be passed from the CPU to the graphics hardware, avoiding the classical CPU bottleneck.

4. Fractal Geometry for Modelling Virtual Landscapes

Fractal geometry can be applied in computer science for modelling landscapes which include mountains, trees, clouds and so forth. An interesting mechanism for generating a kind of fractal mountains, based on recursive subdivision algorithm for a triangle, was developed by Fournier et al. (1982). Here, the midpoints of each side of the triangle are connected, creating four new subtriangles. Figure 5a shows the subdivision of the triangle into four smaller triangle, figure 5b illustrates how the midpoints of the original triangle are perturbed in the y direction (Foley et al., 1997). To perturb these points, can be used the properties of the self-similarity, and the conditional expectation properties of fractional Brownian motion (abbreviated to fBm). The fractional Brownian motion, also known as the "Random Walk Process", was introduced by Mandelbrot and Van Ness in 1968, generalizing the Brownian motion (Bm). FBm basically consists of steps in a random direction and with a step-length that has some characteristic value. The self-similarity is an important property of fBm (if we zoom in on any part of the function we will produce a similar random walk in the zoomed in part). Figure 6 shows a recursive subdivision of an initial polygon using squares. Other polygons can be used to generate the grid (e.g., triangles and hexagons).

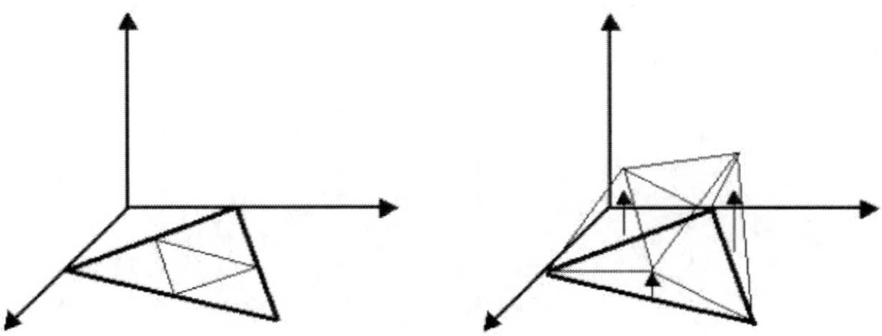

a) b)

Figure 5. The subdivision of a triangle into four smaller triangle a). Perturbation in the y direction of the midpoints of the original triangle b).

This method presents two problems, which can be classified as internal and external consistency problems (Fournier et al., 1982, pp. 374-375). Internal consistency is the reproducibility of the primitive at any position in an appropriate coordinate space and at any level of detail, so the final shape is independent of the orientation of the subdivided triangle. This is satisfied by a Gaussian random number generator which depends on the point's position, so it generates the same numbers in the same order at a given subdivision level. The external consistency refers to the midpoint displacement at shared edges and their direction of displacement. This process, when iterated, generates a deformed grid which represents the wireframe of a surface, an example is shown in figure 6. After the rendering phase (that includes: hidden lines, texture, lighting, and shading information) appears a realistic fractal mountain, as shown in figure 7.

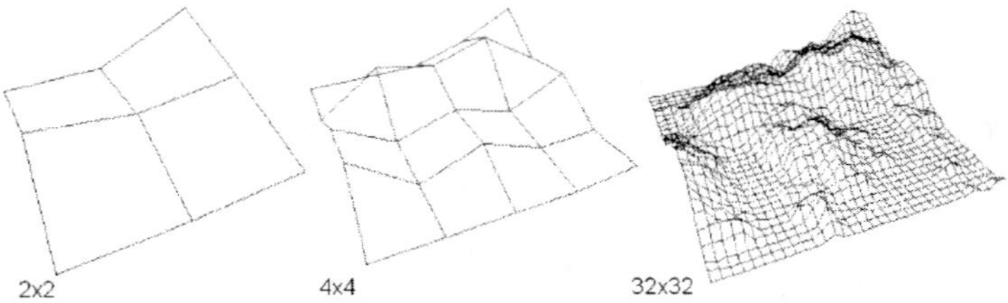

Figure 6. Grid of squares generated by a recursive subdivision and applying the fractional Brownian motion.

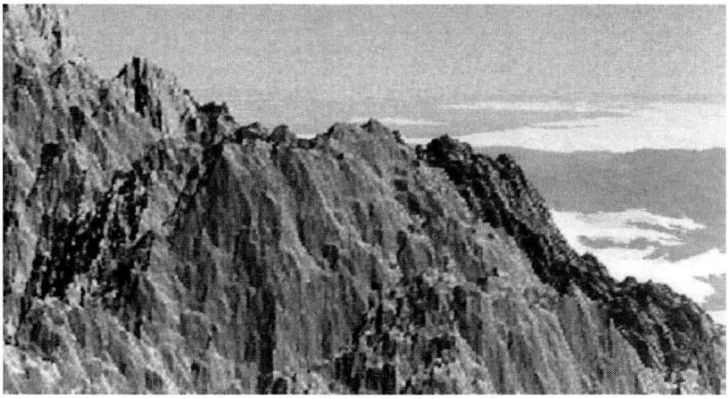

Figure 7. Fractal mountains.

These examples describe how to realize fractal mountains but not their erosion. Interesting techniques which are independent of the terrain creation have been introduced by Musgrave et al. (1989). Their algorithm can be applied to already generated data represented as regular height fields require separate processes to define the mountain and the river system. Prusinkiewicz and Hammel (1993) combined the midpoint-displacement method for mountain generation with the squid-curve model of a non-branching river originated by Mandelbrot (Mandelbrot, 1978; 1979).

This method created one non-branching river as result of context sensitive L-system operating on geometric objects (a set of triangles). Three key problems remained unsolved (i) the river flowed at a constant altitude, (ii) the river flowed in an asymmetric valley, and (iii) the river had no tributaries. Figure 8 shows an example of a squid-curve construction (recursion levels 0–7) (Prusinkiewicz and Hammel, 1993, p. 177).

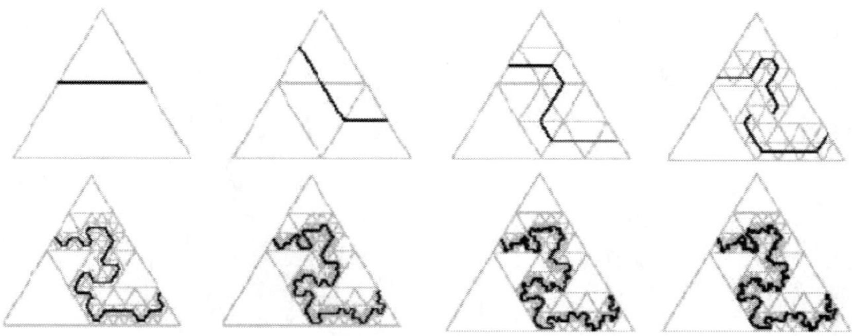

Figure 8. Squid-curve construction (recursion level 0-7).

A method for synthetical terrain erosion, that was based on rewriting process of matrices representing terrain parts, has been introduced by Maràk et al. (1997). They found a rewriting process which was context sensitive. It was defined as a set of productions A → B, where A and B were matrices of numbers of type: N ×N, where N>0.

The terrain parts were rewritten using certain user-defined set of rules which represented an erosion process. The method consisted in three kinds of rewriting process (Maràk et al., 1997; Maràk, 1997). The first is "absolute rewriting" which permitted to erode the objects in predefined altitude.

The second is "rewriting with the reference point" which could erode arbitrary object in any altitude. The third kind of rewriting process permitted to erode some shapes in any scale. Its advantage was that the algorithm could be controlled by some external rules and it could simulate different kinds of erosion (Maràk et al., 1997).

Fractal algorithms can be used in computer graphics to generate complex objects, for example the plant shapes, using Iterated Function Systems. Figure 9 shows a fern leaf created using an IFS that is produced by polygons, in this case: Squares, that are put in one another. The final step of this iterative process shows a fern which has high degree of similarity to real one. L-systems are another kind of fractals used for describing branching trees in a compact format. Originally they were devised to provide a formal description of the development of such simple multicellular organisms. Later on, these systems were extended to describe higher plants and complex branching structures. Smith (1984) was the first to prove that L-systems were useful in computer graphics for describing the structure of certain plants, in his paper: "Plants, Fractals, and Formal Languages". He described that these objects should not be labeled as "fractals" for their similarity to fractals, introducing a new class of objects which Smith called "graftals".

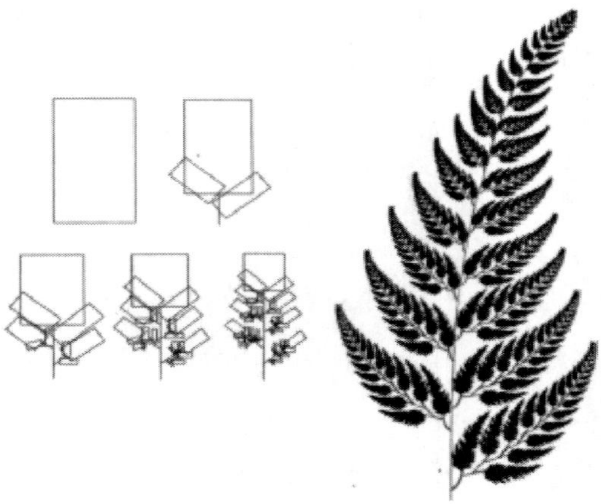

Figure 9. Fern leaf created using the IFS.

This class had of great interest in the Computer Imagery (Smith, 1984; Foley et al., 1997). Figure 10 shows an example of plant-like structures generated after four iterations by bracketed L-systems with the initial string F (angle δ= 22.5°), and the replacement rule F $\rightarrow$FF+[+F-F-F] -[-F+F+F].

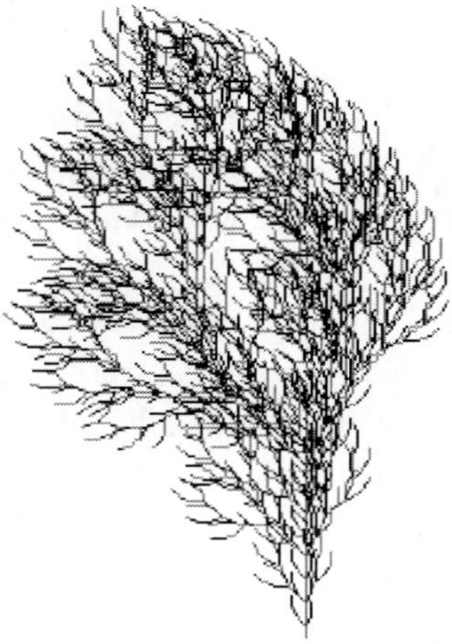

Figure 10. Plant-like structures generated after four iterations by bracketed L-systems.

Fractal algorithms coded in Virtual Reality Modelling Language (VRML) can create virtual mountains and virtual trees, an example is shown in figure 11a. VRML is a 3D graphics language used to create "virtual worlds" networked via the Internet and hyperlinked with the World Wide Web. A virtual world is a computer-based simulated environment generated with fractal algorithms intended for its users to inhabit and interact via avatar (our alter ego in the virtual world). Figure 11b shows a fractal tree generated with simple geometric iterative rules.

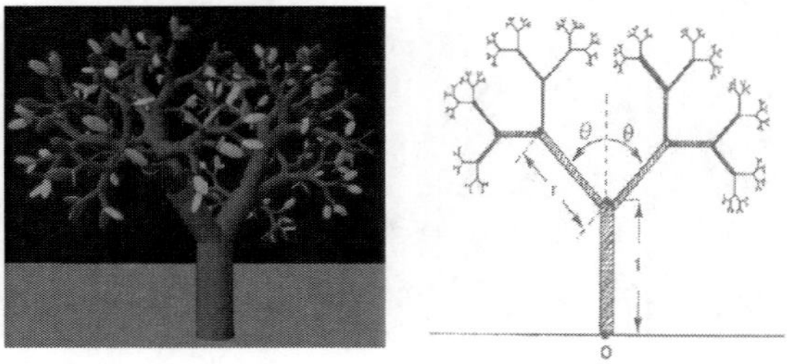

a) b)

Figure 11. Virtual tree realized in VRML using fractal algorithms a). A fractal geometric tree b).

The evolution of the computer graphics techniques and virtual reality technologies, also connected to the fractal algorithms, help to create a new kind of digital arts. Some artists represent a broad range of approaches to installation and virtual reality art (Wands, 2006). For example, Char Davies is a pioneer of this art form. She describes her immersive virtual reality environments *Osmose* (1995) and *Ephémère* (1998) as works "known for their embodying interface, painterly aesthetic and evocation of landscape".

Figure 12 shows the installation space for *Osmose*. Davies and Harrison claim: "*10.5*

immersive virtual environment, produced by Softimage in 1994/95. One of the primary goals of *Osmose* was to push the expressive capabilities of existing 3D tools, to demonstrate that an alternative aesthetic and interactive sensibility is possible for real-time, interactive, 3D computer graphics. *Osmose* was created under the direction of Char Davies, the Director of Visual Research at Softimage.(…) One of Davies' intentions for *Osmose* was to create a space that is "psychically innovating," one in which, to quote Bachelard, participants do not change "place," but change their own nature. *Osmose* was therefore designed to explore the potential of immersive virtual space to allow participants to shed their habitual ways of looking at (and behaving in) the world." (Davies and Harrison, p. 25, 1996).

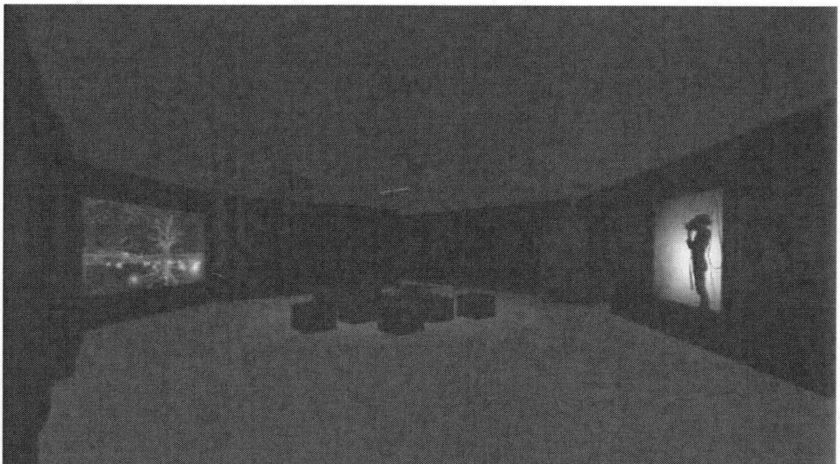

Figure 12. The installation space for *Osmose* (1995). Char Davies/Immersence Inc.and Softimage Inc.©.

Conclusion

This paper has presented some applications of fractal geometry in computer graphics. The self-similarity, important characteristic of the fractal objects, is a unifying concept, and it is an attribute of many laws of nature and innumerable phenomena in the world around us.

In computer graphics, fractals can be applied in different fields, for instance to compress the images using simple algorithms based on Iterated Function Systems, and the image compression is assessed for suitability for spacecraft images. Other application field is to recursively define branching trees, mountains and plant shapes using L-systems and the fractional Brownian motion.

Future trends are oriented to use IFS to generate terrain from real data extracted from geological data base. This is useful in the reconstruction of real terrain and landscapes, for instance in the Geographic Information Systems (GIS) (Guérin et al., 2002; Guérin, and Tosan, 2005). Fractal geometry also offers an alternative approach to conventional planetary terrain analysis. For example, Stepinski et al. (2004) describe Martian terrains, represented by topography based on the Mars Orbiter Laser Altimetry (MOLA) data, as a series of drainage basins. Fractal analysis of each drainage network, computationally extracts some network descriptors that are used for a quantitative characterization and classification of Martian surfaces.

Computer graphics connected to the fractal geometry and to the virtual reality have also given to the digital artists powerful tools and new sources of creative expression (Davies and Harrison, 1996; Thwaites, 2005; Wands, 2006).

References

Barnsley MF. (1988). *Fractals Everywhere*. Boston: Academic Press.

Barnsley MF. (1993). *Fractals Everywhere*. Boston: Academic Press, 2nd edition.

Barnsley MF, Saupe D and Vrscay ER. (Eds.) (2002). *Fractals in Multimedia*. Berlin, Germany: Springer.

Barnsley MF, Jacquin AE, Malassenet F, Reuter L and Sloane AD. (1988). Harnessing chaos for image synthesis. *SIGGRAPH 1988*, pp. 131-140.

Bogomolny A. (1998). *The Collage Theorem*. Retrieved September 1, 2006, from: http://www.cut-the-knot.org/ctk/ifs.shtml.

Davies C and Harrison J. (1996). Osmose: Towards Broadening the Aesthetics of Virtual Reality. *Computer Graphics (ACM SIGGRAPH)*, Vol. XXX (4) (1996) pp. 25-28.

Eglash R. (1999). *African Fractals: Modern Computing and Indigenous Design.* Piscataway, NJ: Rutgers University Press.

Erramilli A, Gosby D and Willinger W. (1993). Engineering for Realistic Traffic: A Fractal Analysis of Burstiness. *Proceedings of ITC Special Congress*, Bangalore, India, 1993.

Fisher Y. (1995). *Fractal Image Compression: Theory and Application*. New York: Springer-Verlag.

Foley JD, van Dam A, Feiner SK and Hughes JF. (1997). *Computer Graphics: Principles and Practice*. Second Edition in C. New York: Addison Wesley.

Fournier A, Fussel D and Carpenter L. (1982). Computer Rendering of Stochastic Models. *Communications of the ACM*, 25, pp. 371-384.

Fractal geometry. (2007). In *Encyclopædia Britannica*. Retrieved February 2, 2007, from Britannica Concise Encyclopedia: http://concise.britannica.com/ebc/article-9364797/fractal-geometry.

Guérin E and Tosan E. (2005). Fractal Inverse Problem: Approximation Formulation and Differential Methods. Lévy-Véhel J and Lutton E. (Eds.*). Fractal in Engineering: New Trends in Theory and Applications*, pp. 271-285. London: Springer.

Guérin E, Tosan E and Baskurt A. (2002). Modelling and Approximation of Fractal Surfaces with Projected IFS Attractors". Novak MM. (Ed.). *Emergent Nature: Patterns, Growth and Scaling in the Science,* pp. 293-303. New Jersey: World Scientific.

Leland WE, Taqqu MS, Willinger W and Wilson DV. (1993). On the Self-Similar Nature of Ethernet Traffic. *Proceedings of the* ACM/SIGCOMM'93, pp. 183-193. San Francisco, CA.

Mandelbrot B. (1975). *Les Objects Fractals. Forme, Hasard et Dimension [Fractal Objects. Form, Chance and Dimension].* Paris, France: Nouvelle Bibliothèque Scientifique Flammaron.

Mandelbrot B. (1982). *The Fractal Geometry of Nature*. San Francisco, CA: W.H. Freeman and Company.

Maràk I. (1997). *On Synthetic Terrain Erosion Modeling*: A Survey. Retrieved March 14, 2007, from: http://www.cescg.org/CESCG97/marak/.

Marák I, Benes B and Slavík P. (1997) Terrain Erosion Model Based on Rewriting of Matrices. *Proceedings of WSCG-97*, vol. 2. pp. 341-351.

Musgrave FK, Kolb CE and Mace RS. (1989). The synthesis and rendering of eroded fractal terrain. *Proceedings of SIGGRAPH '89*, in *Computer Graphics* 23, 3, (pp.41-50), ACM SIGGRAPH, New York.

Nonnenmacher TF, Losa GA, Merlini D and Weibel ER. (Eds.). (1994). *Fractal in Biology and Medicine*. Basel, Switzerland: Birkhauser.

Peitgen H and Saupe D. (1988). *The Science of Fractal Images*. New York: Springer-Verlag.

Prusinkiewicz P and Hammel M. (1993). A Fractal Model of Mountains with Rivers. *Proceeding of Graphics Interface '93*, pp. 174-180.

Prusinkiewicz P and Lindenmayer A. (1990). *The Algorithmic Beauty of Plants*. New York, US: Springer-Verlag. Retrieved September 10, 2007, from: http:// algorithmicbotany.org/papers/abop/abop.pdf.

Sala N. (2006). Complexity, Fractals, Nature and Industrial Design: Some Connections. Novak MM. (Ed.). *Complexus Mundi: Emergent Pattern in Nature*, pp. 171-180. Singapore: World Scientific.

Stepinski TF, Collier ML, McGovern PJ and Clifford SM. (2004). Martian, geomorphology from fractal analysis of drainage networks. *Journal of Geophysical Research*, Vol. 109, nºE2, pp. E02005.1-E02005.12.

Thwaites H. (2005). The Immersant Experience of Osmose and Ephémère. *Proceedings of the 2005 International Conference on Augmented Tele-Existence ICAT '05.* Christchurch, New Zealand, pp. 148-155.

van Wijk JJ and Saupe D. (2004). Image based rendering of iterated function systems. *Computers and Graphics*, 28(6), pp. 937-943.

Vyzantiadou MA, Avdelas AV and Zafiropoulos S. (2007). The application of fractal geometry to the design of grid or reticulated shell structures. *Computer-Aided Design*, Volume 39, issue 1, pp.51-59.

Wands B. (2006). *Art of the Digital Age*. New York, NY: Thames and Hudson Inc.

Wohlberg B, de Jager G. (1999). A Review of the Fractal Image Coding Literature. *IEEE Transactions on Image Processing*, 8(12), pp.1716-1729.

Zhao E and Liu D. (2005). Fractal image compression methods: A review. *ICITA 2005. Third International Conference on Information Technology and Applications*, Volume 1, pp. 756-759.

Section 3. Case Study

Chapter 12

Multidisciplinary Skills in the School of Complexity: Educational Technologies, Human Factor, and Non-Cognitive Skills

Laura Cancellara[*], **Nicoletta Sala, Paola Appeddu, Alessandro Lai and Franco Orsucci**
PM Mind Force Society/MIUR Roma, Italy

Abstract

The SARS-CoV-2 pandemic emergency context has urgently required substantial changes to the socio-educational agencies, requiring an ad hoc reorganization of training strategies. The implementation of innovative technological strategies to support the teaching-learning process requires the attention of new contents and multidisciplinary skills. The digitization of the learning environments proposed in the contribution follow the programmatic lines of an integrated, multidimensional, and complex design approach. The experience of the "Non-cognitive Skills. People, relationships, values" at the GM Angioy Institute and the Wauniversity of Sassari (Italy), experiments with a multi-method approach ESL - Episodes of Situated Learning - (EAS, it refers on the Italian acronym) and focuses attention on not-curricular: artificial intelligence, gamification, robotics, drones, virtual reality. In conclusion, the research is part of the broad interdisciplinary debate about the correlational possibility between traditional "academic" skills, "Digital Skills", the enhancement of "Non-cognitive Skills" with respect to the student's educational success and the achievement of the status of responsible citizen and active participant in social life.

---

[*] Corresponding Author's Email: laura.cancellara@gmail.com.

In: Neuroscience and Technology Transform the Educational Ecosystem
Editors: Franco F. Orsucci and Nicoletta Sala
ISBN: 979-8-88697-157-6

Keyword: non-cognitive skills, educational technologies, ESL, AI, gamification VR, student centered learning, inclusion, equity & human capital

Introduction

The emergency scenario due to the rapid spread of the SARS-CoV-2 pandemic has urgently required substantial changes to the educational and social agencies, imposing a sudden reorganization of socio-relational and institutional networks.

The emerging "VUCA" context, term originally used to describe Volatility, Uncertainty, Complexity, Ambiguity, requires the demanding commitment of educational and training agencies, of a multidisciplinary comparison that must be framed in the perspective of a multidimensional complexity.

Facing this complexity in emergency contexts requires a further systemic analysis.

Conditions characterized by high individual, social and relational vulnerability, require a paradigmatic change: educational and training agencies have an urgent mandate to re-modulate pedagogical strategies and to re-define training interventions attentive to individual and collective "transformative resilience" policies.

It becomes necessarily central to pay attention to psycho-pedagogical research on contextual factors (socio-economic and environmental), which constantly influence individual abilities, psychic, behavioral, socio-relational and emotional processes.

The road map to reach the programmatic address of Objective 4 of the UN 2030 Agenda already provides for the implementation of didactic-educational strategies that are able to face contemporary global challenges. The qualitative objective of guaranteeing equitable educational opportunities and inclusive school cultures, in line with sustainable community development, involves the integration of an adaptive and complex pedagogical approach, attention to "situational expertise" which thus allows the formulation of a planning systemic pedagogical-educational. We are talking about a 'transformational pedagogical device that overlaps in contexts of collective crisis between envisaged and realized, which treasures the experience of lived, through the improvement of the entire educational-training system' (Piceci, Cancellara, 2020).

In recent years, the growing interest of scientific research in the field of education and training in the 'non-cognitive' dimensions of learning, probably encourages us to define them as 'key competences'. These skills are closely related to the dimension of an individual's "transformative resilience." The systematic focus on social and emotional domains and the full realization of students' full development potential was also analyzed by the Programs for International Student Assessment (PISA) and the OECD (Organization for Economic Cooperation and Development).

1. Ecosystemic Factors of Learning

The innovation of the "Learning Compass 2030" program, designed by the Organization for Economic Co-operation and Development (OECD), involves the updating of personalized and digital programs, which define what knowledge, skills, attitudes and values are that students need to realize their potential to be able to contribute to the well-being of their communities and the well-being of the planet.

In this regard, the innovation of the program distinguishes:

- Cognitive and metacognitive skills (Learning to learn)
- Social Skills and Emotional Skills
- Practical and physical skills
- Computational Thinking
- Systems Thinking
- Global Competency

The OECD program classification focuses attention on attitudes and values that are further distinguished into four broad categories:

- *Personal category*- related to the definition of a person's life goals;
- *Social category*- related to interactions and positive relationships with others;
- *Social category*- relating to the promotion of social and institutional cohesion;
- *Human category*- related to the promotion of cultural and global well-being.

The aforementioned approach integrates the dimension of a complexity (figure 1) that gradually embraces itself between the micro, middle and macro levels (individual, interpersonal and social) referring to an interacting ecosystem between the factors that determine learning. It clearly refers to the degree of agency of individuals: all become agents of change and through the relationship and interpersonal interactions, they influence each other. Defining this ecosystem of increasing complexity means directly involving both students and families, teachers, communities, the institutional structure, and the territory.

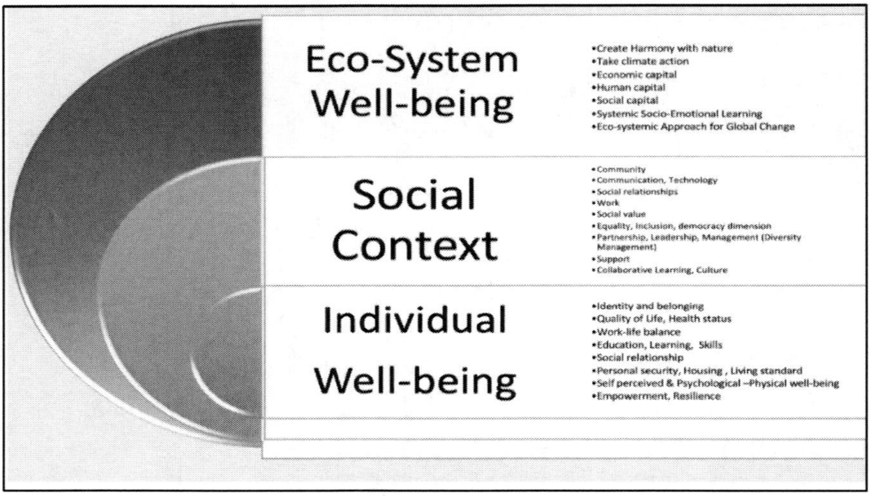

Figure 1. Ecosystems, Social Context and Human Well-being.

1.1. Non-Cognitive Skills and Transformative Learning

The international research landscape refers to "Non-cognitive Skills" to define the set of skills that directly, indirectly, or transversally, condition the learning process and prepare the student, more generally, for the acquisition of the status of adult citizen, responsible and active participant in social life.

Usually, the scientific community focuses on "Non-cognitive Skills" with different interpretations, definitions, and domains, for this reason, there is no well-defined consensual terminology to define them.

Speaking of Non-cognitive Skills therefore means referring to a polysemic term, an umbrella construct that recognizes both theoretical and cognitive knowledge, professional qualifications, behavioral skills, attitudinal traits, motivational systems, interpersonal skills, learning strategies, metacognitive skills and ultimately, is a set of dimensions that influence each other. For this reason, correlations between these traits support the notion of a broad multidimensional definition of non-cognitive abilities (figure 2).

Duckworth & Yeager (2015), in "Measurement Matters: Assessing Personal Qualities Other Than Cognitive Ability for Educational Purposes", in fact, assert the difficulty of being able to conceptually separate the cognitive domains from the non-cognitive domains, since "every aspect of psychological functioning, from perception to personality, it is inherently 'cognitive' to the extent that information processing is involved" (Duckworth & Yeager, 2015).

In conclusion, it is desirable, in this sense, to think of a continuum between "cognitive and non-cognitive" skills.

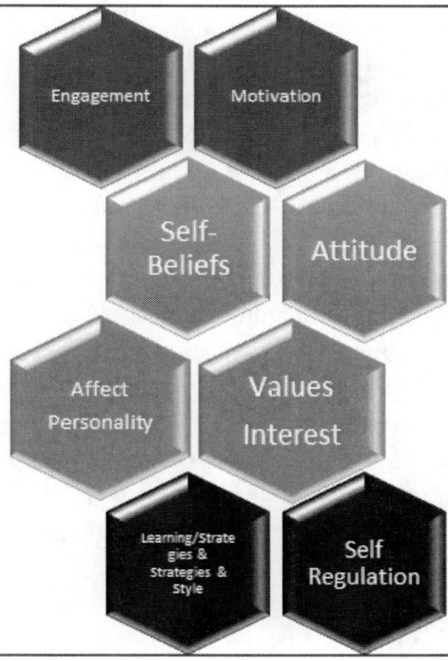

Figure 2. Some examples of Non-Cognitive Grouping in research domains that support multi-dimensionality definition of non-cognitive abilities.

1.2. Non-Cognitive Skills and Human Capital

In 2006, James J. Heckman and the Chicago School (defined as pioneers in recognizing the importance of Non-cognitive Skills) were the first to underline the correlation between skills, self-productivity, and complementarity of investments in human capital.

The paternity of the concept “Skill formation is a life cycle process” (Cunha, Heckman, Lochner, and Masterov, 2006), was the forerunner of a subsequent vast international empirical literature, which focused on research on the formulation of qualitative-quantitative methodologies for measure the effects of the development of Non-cognitive Skills, on a great variety of areas of the person’s life. The operationalization of educational and training strategies based on the acquisition of transversal skills, takes into account data relating to the personality traits, personal goals, motivations and characteristics of each student, which until then had not yet been treated (conscientiousness, intrinsic goal orientation, metacognitive self-regulation). Longitudinal studies, in fact, they deepen the correlation between Cognitive Skills and Non-cognitive Skills in the formulation of the concept of human capital. Becker, GS (1964) defines ‘human capital’ as anything related to the expected return on investment in education.

Even James J. Heckman, former Nobel laureate in economics, known for his studies on human capital, emphasizes that he does not refer to learning by focusing exclusively on mnemonic-cognitive aspects, but to take into account other qualities of the person such as: extroversion, friendliness, conscientiousness, emotional stability and openness to experience.

The current demand of the emerging labor market, in fact, refers to qualities related to coping strategies to cope with stressful situations, self-control, teamwork and conflict management, cognitive flexibility and adaptability to changing situations. Optimism, resilient leadership, systems thinking, and result orientation are also highly sought after skills.

2. Multidimensionality of Non-Cognitive Factors

A systemic, dynamic and non-linear reading of the factors that influence the entire educational context leads us to consider the multidimensionality of Non-cognitive Skills.

Educational factors, personality factors, contextual and situational factors are interrelated in determining the academic performance of each student. When developed in combination, specific skills, such as personal self-efficacy, communication strategies, metacognition skills, intrinsic motivation, seem to positively improve both school learning and educational success, in the direction of a complete development of personal potential. Considering the multifactorial nature of the determinants of learning, there is an increasing need to require educational agencies and trainers/educators for adequate specialized training in dealing with the nature of this complexity.

Although the psychometric measurement of cognitive abilities still remains a determining factor in assessing academic achievement (Cassidy, 2011), there are other non-cognitive learning factors that are defined as indicative predictors of both academic achievement potential and failure risk indices. scholastic (Lauria et al., 2013). To date, these longitudinal studies are further enriched by qualitative analyzes that refer to considering the impact on academic performance, the social context, the role of families (parental engagement), school leadership, institutions and more generally, the territorial stakeholders. Moreover, the OECD working paper "Non-cognitive characteristics and academic achievement in Southeast Asian countries based on Pisa" (2009, 2012, and 2015, OECD Education Working Paper No. 233) introduces "Some specific variables: student demographic background such as gender, home environment often represented by family socio-economic status (SES), school types, and government policies, social structure, and economic development of the country" (OECD, EDU/WKP, 2020-21).

The experiences reported in the following pages are part of the broad interdisciplinary debate that has been developing over the decades regarding the possibility of reconsidering the role between traditional "academic" skills and the enhancement of Non-cognitive Skills and the consequent correlation with educational success and the achievement of the status of adult citizen, responsible and active participant in social life.

At the same time, globalization and the growing digitalization of the contexts in which we live require for all active citizens the acquisition of "Digital skills" that are able to support organizations in managing change.

According to the report "The Future of Jobs 2020" of the WEF (World Economic Forum) in 2030 advanced and increasingly innovative digital skills will be required, which require a mix between acquired technological knowledge and Non-cognitive Skills. The educational agencies, for this reason, have an urgent mandate to contextualize this request and align themselves with the economic world.

3. Case Study 1

Edutainment at the Wauniversity of Sassari (Italy)

Online learning technologies are a major support tool for students' self-study activities. Considering that the latest generations regularly use digital devices to access a vast amount of content of all kinds, that they constantly exploit mobile applications to simplify procedures, solve problems and speed up processes, we can say that the amount of visual, auditory, tactile and emotional stimuli a young person (13-25 years old) is subjected to is far greater than that of someone in the last twenty years. It is no news that a student's average concentration time has dropped dramatically in the last 10 years, partly caused by obsessive use of social networks; the desire to socialise, flirt, gain approval and appreciation, but above all the almost unconscious behaviour of preferring something distant, but considered more fun, stimulating and more entertaining, to something present as an experience with other peers. In many schools, students use smartphones in spite of teachers' lessons and DAD has given them the opportunity to avoid being caught using them, increasing student distraction and decreasing academic performance.

A student spends most of the time on social networks and entertainment platforms.

It could be inferred that digital learning materials, online courses and e-learning platforms are secondary and less effective tools than traditional ones such as books and lectures. Today, it is possible to keep the student's concentration and motivation to study high and at the same time convert the time spent on social networks for activities that are useless for the purpose of acquiring knowledge or skills and exploit them to create study groups and learning communities. This is possible thanks to edutainment, which consists of projects activities, paths and educational projects that contemplate online training technologies, integrate the most widely used entertainment platforms and student engagement strategies adopted by video games.

Wauniversity is a young digital enterprise operating in the training sector, specifically in the support of aspiring health professionals, i.e., students who have to pass university admission selections for medical and health degree courses. The experience gained in 10 years of classroom, online and blended training courses with more than five thousand students of average age 16-22, in the creation of video lessons, books, ebooks, audio books has allowed us to develop a state-of-the-art technology that allows us to considerably enhance the student's academic performance. The design of the e-learning software takes into account numerous characteristics of a student of the latest generation and is based on the WAU! method used in all live courses by Wauniversity teachers and tutors.

The overall Wauniversity training model consists of 5 main pillars

- the student centered model
- the teach-to-learn learning method
- the peer to peer study method
- edutainment
- tutoring

3.1. The Student-Centered Model

This educational model involves the acquisition of knowledge in an active way and also allows for the development of other skills such as creativity, resourcefulness, critical capacity, teamwork etc.

Putting the learner at the center of the learning project also means developing, modifying and improving the same project in which the learner is included thanks to his contribution. They work together with them and with the class to make the learning process more effective and tailor-made. From being an auditor, he becomes a protagonist and therefore lives an active experience of acquiring knowledge through the development and/or enhancement of skills.

This model includes

- an analysis of the student's actual needs.
- a consultation with his teachers and his parents.
- a definition of the competences to be developed and up to which level.
- collegial decisions on how to organize learning activities in the time available.
- collegial decisions on the approaches (to learning, teaching, testing) to be adopted in the chosen activities.
- implementation of a variety of approaches in each training course: since not everyone learns in the same way, teaching and cultural traditions may make the use of different approaches useful.
- transparency: the learner should be informed of what is being asked of him/her, and take an active role in achieving the results);

- flexibility: the student should be able to orient their study plan according to their needs; monitoring and rectifying what does not work.
- mobility (of staff and students, incoming and outgoing) and the systematic exploitation of the benefits it can bring.

Needs, study and behavioral habits, difficulties in achieving objectives, etc., are listened to and deeply understood, thus enabling a friendly and trusting relationship to be established with the child and the class. Above all, it offers the reference teacher the opportunity to understand the individual and overall level of preparation of the class in order to determine the best educational pathway in which to include them.

- The teach-to-learn learning method
- The peer-to-peer study method
- Edutainment
- Tutoring

In May 2021, they launched the first national online WAU! competition in the field of preparation for university selections for medical and health degree courses, with the aim of boosting DAD results, speeding up and simplifying the study of the syllabus to be assessed in the entrance exam and, finally, demonstrating the effectiveness of edutainment and teaching technologies.

(Spot https://www.youtube.com/watch?v=X7hNygUpJeg)

The competition, called Anatomy Experience (https://www.ilsole24ore.com/art/parte-anatomy-experience-prima-competizione-anatomia-realta-virtuale-studenti-tutta-italia-AEafcvE), saw 1000 participants, divided into 100 teams of 10 members, from all over Italy and with an average age of 18.

This training project is structured as follows:

- Students, via the wauniversity.it platform, were able to create their own online team, give it a name and invite other students to join them.
- All teams participated in the launch of the competition and the first activity was to get to know each other through the video conferencing platforms. Most of the teams were composed of members unknown to each other and therefore, in order to respect the Wauniversity training model, the team leader had the task of generating complicity, engagement and mutual trust before entering the competitions. This

process was validated through a test that each member of the team had to pass in order to activate their 'duelist' account, consisting of personal questions about the other members (home town, nickname, school attended, partner's name, etc.);

- Once all accounts were activated, each member took a self-assessment test on the topics of the next lesson, which determined their category. Then the teams participated in the interactive online lesson, given by young medical students (former WAU! students and currently tutors in the live courses) on the topics of the human anatomy syllabus of the exam, with the aid of virtual reality.
- Immediately afterwards, the challenges between teams, called "duel exercises", were opened. Each member of each team, thanks to the profiling obtained from the self-assessment test, challenged the other opponents of the other 99 teams according to their category. The duel exercises consisted of 10 multiple choice quizzes with only one correct answer, all quizzes were commented to quickly provide a complete information sheet of the anatomy topic proposed in the quiz. This allowed the students to immediately understand the error and learn immediately thanks to the high levels of concentration and emotional involvement due to the challenge at hand and the desire to make a contribution, in terms of score, to their team. For each duel won, the winning team gained points for the overall ranking.
- The competition, which lasted 4 days and lasted approximately two hours a day, allowed 1000 students to understand, learn and memorize a quantity of information that in our courses is dealt with in a month's course, in 25 hours of lessons with the teacher and over 40 hours of individual study. Over those four days, the most experienced members of each team consciously adopted the teach-to-learn approach in a peer-to-peer environment, teaching their teammates what they needed to be able to tackle the next challenge, which, after each victory, was more difficult.
- At the end of the fourth day, the top 10 teams faced a final competition that was even more engaging and adrenaline-pumping. The captains chosen by each team faced a head-to-head challenge online (organized in rounds as in football), but this time LIVE, showing themselves live to over 1000 viewers on YouTube https://www.youtube.com/watch?v=uaGwEwDsDMU and the 1000 members of the teams. Each duel consisted of 3 multiple-choice quizzes, different from the previous duel exercises. Just like in the TV programme

"Who wants to be a millionaire" they had aids that could be offered, at the request of the captain, to their teammates.
- The best 3 teams won the competition and received important prizes for their university careers (stethoscope, anatomy atlas, doctor's coat etc.).

Artificial intelligence software, called SELF, was able to profile the students during the competition and propose more effective study activities in order to win the next challenge. The statistics gathered by the LMS WAU! (Learning management system) show that the students' performance improved up to five times more than in previous study sessions, taking into account average scores in mock exams and progress in response speed and mistakes reduction. The best result was at the official entrance exam, four months later, more than 80% of the Anatomy Experience participants correctly answered all the anatomy questions related to the topics of the competition and explained in class by the young tutors.

4. Case Study 2

Non-cognitive skills. People, relationships, values: the Sassari experience (Italy)

The project "Non-cognitive skills. People, relationships, values, was born in 2019 from the experience of the Education and Learning Centre "Gli Improbabili", managed by the San Camillo de Lellis cooperative, and implemented with the collaboration of the Fondazione di Sardegna. The project aims to develop non-cognitive skills among the students of two classes at the of the G. M. Anjoy industrial technical institute in Sassari. In view of the context of socio-cultural high rates of school drop-out - both implicit and explicit - characterizing the Sardinian and territory of Sassari. In view of the socio-cultural context of hardship and the high school drop-out rates - both implicit and explicit - that characterise Sardinia and Sassari, it was decided to define a line of action that would focus on aspects not previously considered by the policies against educational poverty applied so far. For this reason, recent scientific evidence regarding the correlation between the development of NCS and CS has confirmed the need to intervene on the former in order to generate positive outputs on the latter. The project Non-cognitive skills. People, relationships, values; is therefore opening a first glimmer towards a radical change in the way of thinking about the educational system in the region. The context referred to above is characteristic not only of Sardinia but, as is well known, also of central and southern Italy. However, the problem of early school leaving and educational poverty affects the peninsula as a whole when compared with other European countries and especially with other high-income countries or the other G7 powers. However, the reasons that afflict southern Italy and its islands are rooted in years of economic and social backwardness and still weigh on every aspect and indicator that can be studied, including school performance. The aim of the NCS intervention is therefore to find a solution to the deep-rooted educational flaws that have formed over the past decades. The strategy of educational action therefore aims to create a pathway that has as its reference point the creation of stable and lasting relationships both among the subjects that revolve around the education of the children, teachers, parents, other educational realities, the economic and social fabric of the territory, and among the children themselves, at a time when the direct relationship between them is mediated by a society increasingly poor in educational content, continually organized towards an individualistic conception of the person and worsened in terms of knowledge and learning by the increasingly precocious use of digital tools which have made adults and children lose the taste for the beauty of friendship, wonder and knowledge of reality.

The objectives proposed to the project are therefore

- To favor the expression of individual inclinations and potentialitieš;
- To promote experiences of comparison and knowledge with the regional and national economic fabric and national economic fabric;
- To promote a critical spirit;
- Developing greater self-esteem, autonomy, independence and originalitỳ;
- Developing forms of collaboration and shared projects with schools, universitieš, institutions and the business world
- Develop forms of collaboration and shared projects with schools, universitieš, institutions and the economic world;
- Propose forms of dialogue between adults and children;
- Supporting parents in the maturative and evolutionary process of knowledge of school and extracurricular needs.
- Support parents in their maturative and evolutionary knowledge of their child's school and extracurricular needs;
- Developing and supporting the educational role of adults.

The project is in its third year and will end in May 2022. The path of this last year is organized in three phases. The first was the presentation of the initiative to the students and teachers of classes 4A and 4C of the 4A at the IT specialization.

The second stage corresponds to the actual start of the educational pathway, which was officially inaugurated with the seminar held on 29th November 2021 in the Aula Magna of the University of Sassari. During the event the students have been involved not only in the preparation and organization of the meeting but also in its actual implementation. The body of the course consists of scheduled meetings with the students in which non-curricular topics (artificial intelligence, gamification, robotics, drones, virtual reality) were dealt with and are being dealt with by Prof. Nicoletta Sala (associate professor at Institute for Scientific and Interdisciplinary Studies (ISSI) and Research Institute in Arithmetic Physics (IFIA), Switzerland). In this phase, the educational approach is based on Episodes of Situated Learning (EAS, it refers on the Italian acronym). It is a new way for teaching and learning (Rivoltella, 2014; Triacca, Petti, L., & Rivoltella, 2019).

EAS are based on active learning strategies and relate to the three learning domains referred to as knowledge, skills and attitudes. They are based on the following steps:

- a flipped learning approach which starts from research on a certain subject,
- an action on problem solving abilities,
- a classroom discussion engaging students in solving problems in a learn-by-doing environment, and
- a reflective learning approach, where concepts are reworked and restructured using the new media of the communication.

The research of information is done through digital media that are more suitable to digital-natives students. The subsequent experiential paths are carried out by professional coaches, in collaboration with "Associazione Culturale Formore Istruzione" and "Wauniversity" both founded by Alessandro Lai and "Digital Detox Log Out Live Now" by Gavino Puggioni, who develop through the three channels of learning, head (cognitive work), heart (emotional work), hand (learning through movement) and use languages and tools to accompany the development of the perception of the value of realitỳ, living it as a resource of personal experience and possibilitỳ of growth and change. In order to validate this close link between cognitive and non-cognitive growth, indicators prepared by Prof. Franco Orsucci, Professor of Psychology at University College London, will be used, as well as the indicators that were used for the research, carried out by the Foundation for Subsidiarity that gave name and impulse to the project.

The third phase will select the young people who have achieved the best results as a team and individually. The winning team will be able to participate in a qualifying course for the construction and use of drones. The development of this third phase fully involves the mission of the Institute, which is already strongly oriented towards collaboration with local and national companies. It will multidimensional activities will also be proposed to promote the knowledge of the most significant work opportunities that, starting from the methods used in the past, lead to the possibility of innovative future production processes.

In this last part, therefore, the final year students will be involved in orientation activities through moments of confrontation and meeting with the protagonists of the Sardinian entrepreneurial world.

Conclusion

The project evidence operationalized by the experiences lived by the students in recent months are highlighting the usefulness of the new didactic approaches used, ever closer to the real needs of the students. The proposed activities not only positively enhance cognitive skills and strengthen their cognitive impact but also facilitate awareness for the emotional-affective and socio-relational dimensions of the participants.

The development and dissemination of solutions for the creation of digital environments with innovative and sustainable methodologies, offers strategic support that simultaneously supports the training teaching of ministerial paths through experimental activities in the form of laboratory activities, designed ad hoc for students. The "student centered" experience is based on innovative teaching principles and practices that put students at the center: characteristics such as agency, active engagement, promotion of cooperative learning, encourage teachers to empathically tune in to students' motivations, emphasis is placed on individual differences, and training feedback. Talking about educational technologies to a heterogeneous school community, it means dealing with a complex field of study that investigates the process of analysis, design, development, implementation and evaluation of the didactic-training environment, including learning tools. This organization promotes the horizontal interconnection between more character-relational areas and technical-scientific disciplines, which co-create an interacting-hybrid "learning space" (both physical and virtual together). The teaching content is enriched with digital resources, based on virtual and augmented reality, while remaining firmly anchored to the humanizing aspect. Learning spaces that are configured as smart environments for training, real "learning ecosystems" that strengthen the interaction between students-teachers-contents-resources-context. Ultimately, it is to experiment with the modeling of a fair and inclusive teaching, a teaching attentive to the diversity of each and for this, we are talking about personalized learning environments. Carrying out the development of digital teaching projects, digital citizenship, digital education also means, on a broad scale, focusing on initiatives to combat early school leaving and educational poverty. We consider that the enhancement of non-cognitive skills (life skills), designed through the experimentation of innovative teaching activities and aimed at developing transversal skills, should be simultaneous with a teacher training activity. In fact, in order to support students in the learning process and in order to improve the training activities of the teaching staff.

Orienting students means constantly supporting them for the actualization of choices made with awareness, in terms of education and training, also through the teaching of human skills necessary for the construction of one's professional identity, the labor market and active citizenship.

References

Becker, G. S. (1964), *'Human capital theory'*, Columbia, New York 1964.

Duckworth A. L., Yeager D. S. Measurement Matters: Assessing Personal Qualities Other Than Cognitive Ability for Educational Purposes. *Educational Researcher*. 2015; 44(4):237-251. doi: 10.3102/0013189X15584327.

Cassidy, S. (2011). Exploring individual differences as determining factors in student academic achievement in higher education. *Studies in Higher Education*, 37(7), 1–18.

Cunha, F. & Heckman, James J. & Lochner, Lance, (2006). *Interpreting the Evidence on Life Cycle Skill Formation*, Handbook of the Economics of Education, in: Erik Hanushek & F. Welch (ed.), Handbook of the Economics of Education, edition 1, volume 1, chapter 12, pages 697-812, Elsevier.

Cunha, F.; Heckman, J. J.; Lochner, L. J.; Masterov, D. V. (2006). *Interpreting the Evidence on Life Cycle Skill Formation*. In: Hanushek, E. A.; Welch, F., editors. Handbook of the Economics of Education. North- Holland; Amsterdam: 2006. p. 697-812.chap. 12.

Cunha, F., Heckman, J. J. (2007). The Technology of Skill Formation. *American Economic Review*, 97(2), 31-47.

Cunha, F., Heckman, J. J. (2008). Formulating, identifying and estimating the technology of cognitive and noncognitive skill formation. *Journal of Human Resources*, 43(4), 738-782.

Cunha, F., Heckman, J. J., Schennach S. (2010). Estimating the technology of cognitive and noncognitive skill formation. *Econometrica*, 78(3), 883- 931.

Heckman, J. J., Stixrud, J., Urzua, S. (2006). The effects of cognitive and noncognitive abilities on labor market outcomes and social behavior. *Journal of Labor economics*, 24(3), 411-482.

Lauria, E. J. M., Moody, E. W., Jayaprakash, S. M., Jonnalagadda, N., & Baron, J. D. (2013). *Open academic analytics initiative: Initial research findings.* Third Conference on Learning Analytics and Knowledge (LAK 2013), ACM, Leuven, Belgium.

OECD. *Non-Cognitive Characteristics and Academic Achievement In Southeast Asian Countries Based On Pisa 2009, 2012, And 2015*. Oecd Education Working Paper No. 233 Jihyun Lee, The University of New South Wales, Sydney13 October 2020 https://www.oecd.org/officialdocuments/publicdisplaydocumentpdf/?cote=EDU/WKP(2020)21&docLanguage=En.

Piangiamore, G. L., Musacchio, G., & Devecchi, M. (2016). *Episodes of situated learning: natural hazards active learning in a smart school.* In Interactive Learning: Strategies, Technologies and Effectiveness. Ed. NOVA Science Publisher, New York.

Piceci, L.; Cancellara, L.; (2020). *Pedagogy of emergency and vulnerability and Covid-19: psychological aspects and links with technology*; Giornale Italiano di Educazione alla Salute, Sport e Didattica Inclusiva, V. 4, N. 2 (2020): Research and Reflections on Education, Technologies and Psychophysical Well-Being During the Covid-19 Pandemy.

Rivoltella, P. C. (2014). *Episodes of situated learning.* A new way to teaching and learning.

Triacca, S., Petti, L., & Rivoltella, P. C. (2019). Designing and re-designing the e-learning course "Teaching with Episodes of Situated Learning." *Research on Education and Media, 11*(2), 95-100.

About the Editors

Franco Orsucci

Franco Orsucci received his first degree in Medicine and second degree in Psychiatry at La Sapienza University in Rome (Italy). He has been a researcher at the Italian National Research Council. He was also a research fellow at the London University College. He is visiting Professor a UCl, Fellow of the European Academy of Sciences and Arts, Senior Consultant at the NHS, and founder and editor of Chaos and Complexity Letters International Journal of Dynamical System Research (Nova Science, New York). His important books are Changing Mind, Transitions in Natural and Artificial Environments (World Scientific, Singapore, 2002) and Bioethics in Complexity (Imperial College Press, London, 2004). He has also published more than 100 scientific articles on neuroscience and cognitive science.

Nicoletta Sala

Nicoletta Sala received the degree in Physics ("Laurea") at the University of Milan (Italy). Two Masters in Communication and Mass media. Ph-D in Communication and Information Sciences (cum laude) at University of Lugano (Switzerland). She is professor in Information Technology and Electronics Sciences. She taught at Academy of Architecture (Mendrisio, Switzerland), European School of Economics (Italy) and University of Insubria (Varese, Italy). She is professor and scholar at Institute for Scientific and Interdisciplinary Studies (ISSI, Switzerland) and Research Institute in Arithmetic Physics (IRFIA, Switzerland). She is founder and editor of Chaos and Complexity Letters (Nova Science, New York), since 2005. Her last books are: Cappellato G. and Sala N. (2018) Chaos and Complexity in the Arts and Architecture: Research in Progress, Nova Science, New York, and Cappellato G. and Sala N. (2019) Connections Between Mathematics, the Arts and Architecture, Nova Science, New York.

Index

L

M

N

O

P

Q

R

S